Handbook of
Orthopedic
Terminology

Ray F. Kilcoyne, M.D.
Professor of Radiology
Health Science Center
University of Texas
at San Antonio

Edward L. Farrar, M.D.
Orthopedic Surgeon
Wenatchee, Washington

Illustrations by:
Dinah Wilson, B.S.

CRC Press
Boca Raton   Ann Arbor   Boston

Library of Congress Cataloging-in-Publication Data

Kilcoyne, R. F.
Handbook of orthopedic terminology / authors, Ray F. Kilcoyne and
  Edward L. Farrar.
       p.   cm.
  An expanded version of: Handbook of radiologic orthopaedic terminology.
  Includes bibliographical references.
  Includes index.
  ISBN 0-8493-3537-X
  1. Radiography in orthopedics — Terminology.   I. Farrar, Edward.
II. Kilcoyne, R. F. Handbook of radiologic orthopaedic terminology.
III. Title.
  [DNLM: 1. Fractures — terminology.   2. Orthopedics — terminology.
WE 15 K48ha]
RD734.5.R33k54   1991
617.3 — dc20
DNLM/DLC
for Library of Congress   90-2565
                                                              CIP

This book represents information obtained from authentic and highly regarded sources. Reprinted material is quoted with permission, and sources are indicated. A wide variety of references are listed. Every reasonable effort has been made to give reliable data and information, but the author and the publisher cannot assume responsibility for the validity of all materials or for the consequences of their use.

All rights reserved. This book, or any parts thereof, may not be reproduced in any form without written consent from the publisher.

Direct all inquiries to CRC Press, Inc., 2000 Corporate Blvd., N.W., Boca Raton, Florida, 33431.

© 1991 by CRC Press, Inc.

International Standard Book Number 0-8493-3537-X

Library of Congress Card Number 90-2565
Printed in the United States

PREFACE

This handbook is an extension of our earlier work, *Handbook of Radiologic Orthopaedic Terminology*, which was published by Year Book Medical Publishers. Since the release of that text we have received helpful advice and criticism from friends and reviewers. We have tried to respond to those with the production of this expanded handbook.

As in the case of the earlier work, our aim was to provide a ready reference for the radiologist at the work station so that the reporting of orthopedic radiographic studies could be more comprehensive and thus provide a useful service to the referring orthopedic surgeon. Other practitioners who come in contact with orthopedic terminology may also find this book to be of help.

We wish to thank Dinah Stone Wilson for the excellent line drawings, which depict all of the specific anatomic features that are described. Because of the brevity of the text, the entire "message" depends upon the quality of the illustrations. We also want to thank Robert Grant, the late John Snyder, and Barbara Caras of CRC Press, who have encouraged us in undertaking this project.

As always, we would be grateful if readers would communicate with us regarding the usefulness of this text.

R. F. Kilcoyne, M.D.
San Antonio, Texas

Edward L. Farrar, M.D.
Wenatchee, Washington

CREDITS

The following figures were drafted for the *Handbook of Radiologic Orthopaedic Terminology* by R. F. Kilcoyne and Edward Farrar (© 1986 Year Book Medical Publishers, Chicago) and are reprinted by permission.

Figures 2.1–15, 2.17a-d; 4.2–4; 5.1, 5.4–10; 6.5–7, 6.9–12, 6.16–19; 7.1–9, 7.13-20; 8.1–15; 9.1–3, 9.4 (parts 2 & 3); 10.1–8, 10.10, 10.13–14, 10.17–18; 11.1–15.

TABLE OF CONTENTS

1

GLOSSARY OF FRACTURES
WITH EPONYMS
OR DESCRIPTIVE
TERMINOLOGY

INTRODUCTION

The use of eponyms in describing fracture anatomy and relation-ships predates the discovery of X-rays in 1895. Some of the terms have acquired new meanings through the years, and some are controversial. The radiologist should be aware of the existence of these terms so that he or she can understand orthopedic shorthand. Many times it is better in the radiographic report to avoid the use of eponyms and to describe the fracture pattern instead.

Anterior malleolus fracture — Uncommon fracture of the anterolateral margin of the distal tibia at the site of attachment of the anterior tibiofibular ligament. This fragment is also known as the tubercle of Chaput.

Archer's shoulder — Recurrent posterior subluxation or dislocation of the shoulder.

Aviator's astragulus — A variety of fractures of the talus that include compression fractures of the neck, fractures of the body or posterior process, or fractures with dislocations.

Backfire — See Chauffeur fracture.

Bado — A classification of Monteggia-type fractures based on the direction of dislocation of the radial head.

Bankart — A detached fragment from the anteroinferior margin of the glenoid rim. It is seen with anterior shoulder dislocations.

Barton — Intraarticular fracture of the rim of the distal radius. It may involve either the dorsal or volar rim.

Baseball finger — Hyperflexion injury to the distal interphalangeal joint, often associated with a dorsal avulsion fracture of the base of the distal phalanx. It is also called *dropped* or *mallet finger.*

Basketball foot — Subtalar dislocation of the foot.

Bennett — Intraarticular avulsion fracture subluxation of the base of the first metacarpal. The fracture produces a small volar lip fragment that remains attached to the trapezium and trapezoid by means of the strong volar oblique ligament while the shaft fragment is displaced by proximal muscle pull.

Bennett, "Reverse" — Intraarticular fracture subluxation of the base of the fifth and/or fourth metacarpal.

Boot-top — Ski-boot fracture of the midportion of the distal one third of the tibia and fibula.

Bosworth — Fracture of the distal fibula with locking of the proximal fibular fragment behind the tibia.

Boutonniere deformity — Hyperflexion of a proximal interphalangeal joint of a finger due to disruption of the central slip of the extensor tendon.

Boxer — Fracture of the neck of the fifth metacarpal with dorsal angulation, and often volar displacement of the metacarpal head.

Boyd — A classification of intertrochanteric and subtrochanteric hip fractures.

Bucket handle — Vertical shear fracture of the anterior pubis and the opposite ilium.

Buckle — See Torus fracture.

Bumper — Compression fracture of the lateral tibial plateau often associated with avulsion of the medial collateral ligament of the knee. It is also called fender fracture.

Bunionette — An abnormally prominent fifth metatarsal head caused by lateral bending of the fifth metatarsal in combination with a dumbbell-shaped metatarsal head.

Bunkbed — Intraarticular fracture of the base of the first metatarsal in a child.

Burst — Severe comminution of a vertebral body, usually secondary to axial loading, sometimes with a rotatory component. Frequently there is a sagittal fracture through the body plus fractures in the posterior elements. This pattern is often seen with unstable spinal fractures.

Butterfly fragment — Comminuted wedge-shaped fracture that has split off from the main fragments. This implies a high velocity of trauma from a direction opposite the fragment.

Chance — Flexion distraction injury that results in compression of the vertebral body. Posteriorly there may be ligament disruption without fracture, and the disc-anulus complex may be disrupted. Alternatively, there may be transverse non-comminuted fractures of the vertebral body and neural arch. It is also known as lap-type seat belt fracture.

Chaput — Eponym for the anterior tubercle of the distal tibia where the anterior tibiofibular ligament attaches.

Chauffeur — Intraarticular oblique fracture of the styloid process of the distal radius. It is also called backfire, lorry driver, or Hutchinson fracture.

Chisel — Intraarticular fracture of the head of the radius extending distally about 1 cm from the center of the articular surface.

Chopart — Fracture-dislocation of the talonavicular and calcaneocuboid joints. It is derived from Chopart's description of an amputation through these midtarsal joints.

Clay-shoveler — Avulsion fracture of the spinous process of one or more of the lower cervical or upper thoracic vertebrae, most commonly at C-7. More than one vertebra may be involved.

Coach's finger — Dorsal dislocation of a proximal interphalangeal joint.

Colles — Transverse fracture of the distal radial metaphysis proximal to the joint with dorsal displacement of the distal fragment and volar angulation. The ulnar styloid may also be fractured. It is also known as *Pouteau fracture.*

Colles, "reverse" — See Smith fracture.

Corner sign — Metaphyseal fracture fragment secondary to epiphyseal dislocation and resulting epiphyseal plate fracture (Salter-Harris II fracture).

Cotton — Trimalleolar ankle fracture with the posterior tibial fragment displaced posteriorly and superiorly.

Danis-Weber (AO) — A classification of ankle fractures based on the location of the fibular fracture in relation to the syndesmosis and to the horizontal tibiotalar joint.

Dashboard — Fracture of the posterior rim of the acetabulum caused by impact through the knee driving the femoral head against the acetabulum. It is frequently associated with a posterior cruciate ligament injury, a femoral shaft fracture, or patellar fracture.

Denis — A classification of spinal fractures with instability based on a "three column" hypothesis.

De Quervain disease — Stenosing tenosynovitis of the first dorsal compartment of the wrist.

Desault — Various dislocations of the distal radioulnar joint.

Descot — Fracture of the "third malleolus," i.e., the posterior lip of the tibia.

Die punch — Depression fracture of the lunate fossa of the distal radius, allowing proximal migration of the lunate. Also called *lunate load fracture.*

Dome — Fracture involving the weight-bearing surface of the acetabulum or the upper articular surface of the talus.

Dropped — See Baseball finger.

Dupuytren — Fracture of the fibula 2 1/2 in. above the tip of the lateral malleolus caused by a pronation-external rotation injury. It is associated with tear of the tibiofibular ligaments and the deltoid ligament (or fracture of the medial malleolus).

Duverney — Isolated fracture of the iliac wing.

Essex-Lopresti — Comminuted fracture of the head of the radius with dislocation of the distal radioulnar joint.

Extra octave — Salter-Harris II fracture of the fifth proximal phalanx of the hand (with ulnar deviation).

Fender — See Bumper fracture.

Fielding — Classification of subtrochanteric hip fractures based on distance from the lesser trochanter (I–III).

Freiberg's infraction — Flattening of the second metatarsal head. Freiberg felt that this was due to fracture and not osteochondrosis.

Frykman — Classification of distal radius fractures based on involvement of the radiocarpal/radioulnar joints with or without ulnar styloid fracture.

Galeazzi — Fracture of the radius at the junction of the middle and distal thirds with associated dislocation of subluxation of the distal radioulnar joint. Also called a *reverse Monteggia fracture.*

Gamekeeper — Partial or total disruption of the ulnar collateral ligament at the metacarpophalangeal joint of the thumb. It may also have an avulsion fracture from the base of the proximal phalanx.

Garden — Classification of femoral neck fractures. Types I, II, III, and IV are based on the amount of displacement of the femoral neck that is present.

Gosselin — A V-shaped fracture of the lower third of the tibia that extends distally into the tibial plafond.

Greenstick — Incomplete fracture of the shaft of a long bone with disruption on the tension side and plastic deformation on the compression side, resulting in angulation and bowing.

Hangman — Traumatic spondylolisthesis with fracture through the pedicles or lamina of C-2 secondary to a distraction-extension force.

Hawkins — A classification of talar fracture-dislocations.

Hawkins sign — Radiolucent line in the dome of the talus indicating that the talus fracture will heal without osteonecrosis. This subchondral osteoporosis can only develop if the blood supply of the talus is intact.

Henderson — Trimalleolar fracture of the ankle.

Hill-Sachs — Posterolateral defect of the humeral head due to anterior shoulder dislocation and "implosion" fracture.

Hill-Sachs, "reverse" — Anterior defect of the humeral head secondary to posterior shoulder dislocation.

Hip pointer — An impaction fracture of the superior iliac wing.

Hoffa — Coronal fracture of the medial femoral condyle.

Holstein-Lewis — Fracture of the humerus at the junction of the middle and distal thirds where the radial nerve is tethered by the lateral intermuscular septum. Thus, it is associated with radial nerve palsy.

Horseback rider's knee — Dislocation of the fibular head due to a bump against the gatepost.

Hutchinson — See Chauffeur fracture.

Insufficiency — A stress fracture through pathologic bone (usually osteoporotic). Commonly seen in the pelvic ring or femoral neck.

Jefferson — Burst fracture of the ring of the atlas, with fractures both anterior and posterior to the facet joints. It is secondary to an axial load on top of the head. There are usually four breaks in the ring and lateral spread of the lateral masses.

Jockey cap patella — Lateral spurring and deformity of the patella due to chronic lateral subluxation.

Jones — A term sometimes applied to both extra- and intraarticular fracture of the base of the fifth metatarsal. The fracture, which Jones himself experienced, was about 2 cm distal to the tuberosity.

Jumper's knee — Patellar tendinitis.

Juvenile tillaux — Intraarticular fracture of the anterolateral part of the distal tibial epiphysis (tubercle of Chaput) in children aged 12–14 years. This is a Salter-Harris III fracture.

Kocher — Intraarticular fracture of the capitellum of the humerus.

Kohler — Fracture of the tarsal navicular with aseptic necrosis (in children).

Lauge-Hanson — A classification of ankle fractures, based on the mechanism of injury.

Laugier — Fracture of the trochlea of the humerus.

Lead pipe — A combination of greenstick and torus fractures of the forearm.

Le Fort (fibula) — Avulsion fracture of the fibular attachment of the anterior tibiofibular ligament.

Lisfranc — Fracture-dislocation through the tarsometatarsal joints, commonly associated with disruption of the second tarsometatarsal joint and lateral dislocation of the second through fifth tarsometatarsal joints. It may also show other patterns of tarsometatarsal disruption. It is named for Lisfranc's description of an amputation through the tarsometatarsal joints.

Little-leaguer's elbow — Avulsion of the medial epicondyle of the elbow secondary to valgus stress.

Lorry driver — See Chauffeur fracture.

Lunate load — See Die punch fracture.

Maisonneuve — Fracture of the proximal third of the fibula with tear of the distal tibiofibular syndesmosis and the interosseous membrane. It may also have fracture of the medial malleolus or tear of the deltoid ligament.

Malgaigne (of humerus) — Extension-type supracondylar fracture.

Malgaigne (of pelvis) — Fracture-dislocation of one side of the pelvis. This is an unstable injury with two vertical fractures produced by a vertical shear force. The anterior fracture is in the superior and inferior rami of the pubis, and the posterior fracture or dislocation is in the ilium, the sacrum, or the sacroiliac joint. This makes the lateral fragment (containing the acetabulum) unstable.

Mallet — See Baseball finger.

March — Stress or fatigue fracture of the metatarsals. (Other bones may have stress or fatigue fractures.)

Mason — A classification of radial head fractures based on the amount of articular surface involved (I–IV).

Mechanical bull thumb — Fracture at the base of the first metacarpal.

Midnight — Oblique fracture of the proximal phalanx of the fifth toe.

Monteggia — Fracture of the proximal third of the ulna with an anterior dislocation of the radial head. Other types of ulnar shaft fractures and radial head dislocations are sometimes included. The classification of these fractures of Bado is I: ulnar shaft fracture with anterior radial head dislocation; II: ulnar shaft fracture with lateral radial head dislocation; III: ulnar shaft fracture with posterior radial head dislocation; IV: both forearm bones fractured with radial head dislocation.

Monteggia, "reverse" — See Galeazzi fracture.

Montercaux — Fracture of the fibular neck associated with diastasis of the ankle mortise.

Moore — Colles fracture of the distal radius with fracture of the ulnar styloid and dorsal subluxation of the distal ulna.

Mouchet — Fracture of the capitellum of the humerus.

Nightstick — Single bone fracture of the ulnar shaft due to a direct blow without disruption of the interosseous membrane or either of the radioulnar joints.

Nursemaid elbow — Dislocation of the radial head in a toddler with an intact annular ligament. It is difficult to prove with X-ray because the radial head may not be ossified. The dislocation may be reduced by supination during the X-ray examination.

Osgood-Schlatter's lesion — Initially described as an osteochondrosis; a chronic tension failure at the site of attachment of the patellar tendon on the tibial tuberosity.

Parachute jumper —Anterior dislocation of the fibular head.

Paratrooper — Fracture of the distal tibial and fibular shafts.

Pauwels —Fracture of the proximal femoral neck. Types I, II, and III designate the angle of the fracture.

Petit — Osteoporotic stress fracture of the femoral neck in the elderly.

Piedmont — Oblique distal radius fracture without disruption of the distal radioulnar joint. It is difficult to control by closed means. It was described at a Piedmont Orthopaedic Society Meeting.

Pilon — Comminuted, intraarticular fracture of the distal tibia with a long oblique component, secondary to axial loading and impaction of the talus into the tibial plafond.

Pipkin — A classification of femoral head fractures based on the amount of head fractured (I–III).

Plafond — Fracture through the articular surface (plafond = Greek for *ceiling)* of the distal tibia.

Posada — Transcondylar fracture of the distal humerus with anterior flexion of the condylar fragment and posterior dislocation of the radius and ulna.

Pott — Usually a misnomer applied to bimalleolar fractures of the ankle; originally used to describe an abduction injury with fracture of the distal fibula 2–3 in. above the ankle and disruption of the medial ankle ligaments (or avulsion of the medial malleolus).

Pouteau — See Colles fracture.

Pulled elbow — See Nursemaid elbow.

Ring — Fracture involving at least two parts of the pelvic circumference.

Rolando — Severely comminuted Y- or T-shaped fracture through the base of the first metacarpal.

Salter-Harris — A classification of growth plate injuries. State I = epiphyseal plate fracture; II = I + metaphyseal fragment (Thurston-Holland sign); III = I + epiphyseal fragment; IV = II + III; V = I + severe comminution.

Seat belt fracture — See Chance fracture.

Segmental fracture — Fracture dividing the long bone into several segments.

Segond — Avulsion fracture of the lateral tibial condyle at the site of attachment of the lateral capular ligament. This fracture is posterior to the attachment of the iliotibial tract on Gerdy's tubercle. It is often associated with anterior cruciate ligament injury.

Shepherd — Fracture of the lateral tubercle of the posterior process of the talus (which may simulate an os trigonum).

Sideswipe — Comminuted fracture of the distal humerus. It may include fracture of the radius and ulna.

Sinding-Larsen-Johansson injury — Chronic tension failure at the chondroosseous junction of the distal pole of the patella.

Sinegas — A classification of acetabular fractures.

Ski boot — See Boot-top fracture.

Ski pole — Fracture of the base of the first metacarpal. It may be intraarticular.

Smith — Transverse fracture of the distal radial metaphysis with anterior displacement of the distal fracture fragment. The fracture may be intraarticular. It is also called reverse Colles or reverse Barton or Smith-Goyrand fracture.

Sprinter — Fracture of the anterior-superior or the anterior-inferior spine of the ilium with a fragment of bone being avulsed by sudden muscular pull.

Stieda — Avulsion fracture of the medial femoral condyle at the origin of the tibial collateral ligament. It is also used in the term *Pelligrini-Stieda disease,* which describes ossification in the tibial collateral ligament at the margin of the medial femoral condyle from chronic trauma.

Straddle — Bilateral fractures of the superior and inferior pubic rami.

Swan neck deformity — Hyperextension of the proximal interphalangeal joint of the finger secondary to disruption of the volar plate or contracture of the intrinsic muscles.

Tailor's bunion — See Bunionette.

Teardrop — Comminuted vertebral body fracture with a displaced anterior fragment. It is caused by an axial compression force with flexion of the midcervical spine. The same term sometimes is applied to an extension injury. It implies possible instability with posterior displacement of the vertebral body producing spinal cord damage.

Thomas-Epstein — A classification of posterior hip fracture-dislocations.

Thurston-Holland — A metaphyseal fracture "sign" in association with an epiphyseal fracture (Salter-Harris II fracture).

Tillaux — Triad of deltoid rupture or medial malleolar avulsion, fibular fracture 5–6 cm above the ankle joint, and avulsion of the tibial tubercle with diastasis of the syndesmosis. Also see Juvenile tillaux.

Toddler — A nondisplaced fracture of the shaft of the tibia in an infant who has recently begun to walk. Usually spiral in nature and thought to be due to a twisting injury.

Tongue — Horizontal fracture of the posterior-superior surface of the calcaneus.

Torus — Compression fracture of a long bone in or near the metaphysis. It is usually an incomplete fracture and occurs in young children. It is derived from the Greek term for the "bulge" in an architectural column.

Trimalleolar — Fracture of the medial and lateral malleoli and the posterior articular lip of the distal tibia. The term was coined by Henderson.

Triplane — Fracture of the distal tibia involving the growth plate in early adolescence. The fracture lines are in the sagittal, coronal, and axial planes. The three fragments are tibial shaft, antero-lateral epiphysis, and the remaining epiphysis and posterior metaphyseal fragment. This complex fracture pattern is basically a Salter-Harris type II–IV fracture.

Turf toe — Hyperextension injury to the capsule of the first metatarsal phalangeal joint.

Wagon wheel — Traumatic separation of the distal femoral epiphysis.

Wagstaff-Le Fort —Avulsion of the distal fibula at the site of attachment of the anterior inferior tibiofibular ligament.

Walther — Transverse ischioacetabular fracture. The fracture line passes through the ischiopubic junction, the acetabular cavity, and the ischial spine.

Weber — See Danis-Weber (AO).

Wilson — Fracture of the volar plate of the middle phalanx of a finger.

Zickel — A classification of subtrochanteric fractures of the proximal femur based on angulation and/or comminution of the fracture.

REFERENCES

Rang, M. *Anthology of Orthopaedics.* (Edinburgh: E. & S. Livingstone, 1968).

Rockwood, C. A., Jr. and D. P. Green, Eds. *Fractures in Adults. Fractures in Children.* (Philadelphia: Lippincott, 1984).

Schultz, R. J. *The Language of Fractures.* (Huntington, NY: Robert E. Kreiger, 1976).

2

ORTHOPEDIC TERMINOLOGY FOR FRACTURES AND FRACTURE TREATMENT

INTRODUCTION

The radiology report is the unbiased, objective description of the patient's condition. It should convey an accurate report of the fracture pattern and alignment, the status of healing, and the type of internal or external fixation. It has immense medical and legal implications and deserves more than a simple statement about "satisfactory position and alignment".

The purpose of this book is to enable the radiologist to communicate effectively with the orthopedic surgeon. We have attempted to provide a vocabulary that is current and widely accepted among orthopedic surgeons. However, we realize that complete agreement on terminology is unlikely and that differences will occur in various practices.

For more in-depth discussion related to fractures and fracture treatment, the reader is directed to the references at the end of this chapter.

Fracture Pattern and Location

1. Complete or incomplete fracture
    Describes the extent of fracture line across the width of the bone.

2. Closed or open fracture
    a. Closed (simple) fractures do not communicate with the external environment through broken skin.
    b. Open (compound) fractures do communicate with the external environment through broken skin produced by:
        • puncture from within outward by a bony fragment (usually grade I)
        • penetration of the skin by external injury that proceeds to fracture of the underlying bone (usually grade II)
        • crush or avulsion injury with massive soft tissue destruction in association with the fracture (usually grade III)

3. Type of fracture line
    a. Transverse: the line is transverse to the long axis of the bone.
    b. Oblique: the line is oblique to the long axis of the bone.
    c. Spiral: the line is spiral about the long axis of the bone.
    d. Comminuted: multiple fracture lines with three or more fragments. Certain of these may have a Y or T pattern.
        Comminuted fractures are usually associated with higher energy injury and greater soft tissue trauma.
    e. Segmental: fracture lines at two or more levels in the same bone.
    f. Impacted: the collapse of one fragment into another, usually with such apposition that the fracture has some inherent stability.

4. Location
    a. Intraarticular: fracture into a joint cavity.
    b. Proximal or distal shaft (metaphyseal).
    c. Midshaft (diaphyseal).
    d. Epiphyseal plate: through the growth cartilage in children.

5. Pathologic fracture
    A fracture through an area of diseased or weakened bone, often secondary to an underlying process that has altered the structure of the bone.

6. Special cases
    a. Segmental loss: implies that a portion or segment of a bone is actually missing.

b. Fractures involving the epiphysis of a growing bone.
c. Incomplete fractures: a type of fracture in a growing bone that is characterized by fracture of the cortex under tension and bending of the opposite cortex (torus or greenstick fracture or plastic bowing).

RELATIONSHIP OF THE FRACTURE FRAGMENTS TO EACH OTHER

1. ***Displacement*** — describes the apposition of the fracture fragments. These may show a wide range of displacement. (Described as mm or % displacement.)

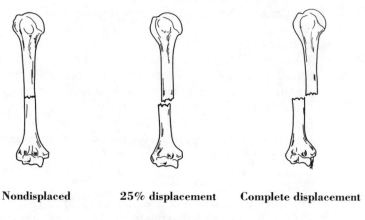

Nondisplaced   25% displacement   Complete displacement

FIGURE 2.1.

2. ***Shortening*** — describes the amount of overlap of fracture fragments.

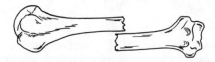

FIGURE 2.2. Shortening of fractures.

3.   ***Angulation*** — describes the deformity that results from a change in the long axis of the fracture fragments measured as a difference in angle from the normal alignment. The apex of the acute angle formed describes the direction of angulation, e.g., "apex volar angulation".

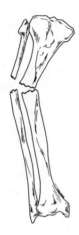 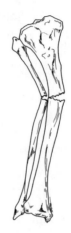

Varus — angulation of the distal fragment toward the midline.   **Valgus — angulation of the distal fragment away from the midline.**

FIGURE 2.3.

4.   ***Rotation*** — describes the change in position that occurs when one fragment rotates with respect to another.

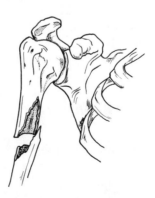

FIGURE 2.4. Fracture rotation.

Fracture Treatment

Reduction of the fracture into anatomic alignment is the goal of treatment. However, it is not always possible or desirable to employ strenuous methods in an attempt to attain this. Imperfect apposition of the fracture fragments can be accepted, but usually imperfect alignment cannot. Problems resulting from displacement or angulation at the fracture site will vary considerably depending upon the site of fracture, the type of fracture, and the age of the patient.

Immobilization is used to prevent displacement or angulation of the fragments, to prevent movement that might interfere with union, and to relieve pain.

Assessment of Healing

Factors that relate to how well healing is progressing include:

Formation of callus — radiodense periosteal and endosteal lines bridging a fracture gap.

Primary bone union — healing of a fracture by trabecular new bone (due to perfect apposition) without callus formation.

Early union — appearance of a trabecular pattern across a fracture line.

Established union — cortical structure and remodeling begin to appear.

Remodeling — reorganization of trabeculae along lines of weight-bearing stress.

Fibrous union — clinically stable, pain-free fracture line without radiographic evidence of union

Nonunion — (atrophic or hypertrophic) failure of a fracture to unite. This is a clinical diagnosis rather than a radiologic diagnosis, although established hypertrophic nonunion is easy to detect radiographically.

The Radiologist's Report

Use of standardized terminology, such as described in this chapter and in the references, will help eliminate misunderstanding and prevent "overreading" and "underreading" of the findings. The description should be limited to anatomic and physiologic terms regarding fracture configuration, alignment, degree of healing, etc. At all costs, terms of a qualitative nature, such as *satisfactory, good* and *worse than expected*, must be avoided, since the radiograph is only one of many factors that help determine the ultimate fate of a fracture and its treatment.

METHODS OF REDUCTION

1. Closed manipulation: with or without plaster immobilization
2. Mechanical traction: with or without external fixation pins
3. Internal fixation
4. External fixation

PRINCIPLES OF INTERNAL FIXATION

1. Anatomic reduction of fracture fragments

2. Fixation with screws, plates, pins, or intramedullary rods. If percutaneous placement of these is used to stabilize a fracture without actually opening the fracture site through a distal skin incision, this procedure is referred to as "closed reduction with percutaneous pinning".

3. Types of internal fixation
   a. Compression screws

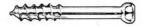

FIGURE 2.5. Cancellous bone screws: Interfragmental compression acts on the whole fracture surface and is achieved by means of a smooth shank proximally and coarse threads distally that provide lag screw fixation. The threads of the screw should never cross the fracture line or the compression effect is lost.

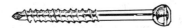

FIGURE 2.6. Malleolar screws: These are used as a cancellous screw but with a self-tapping thread so that they may be used in metaphyseal bone without pre-drilling.

   b. Cortical screws

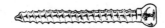

FIGURE 2.7. Cortical screws: Fully threaded and designed for use in cortical bone.

c. Plates

  1. ***Neutralization plate***— used in addition to interfragmentary screws. Such a plate protects the screw fixation by neutralizing torsional, shear, and bending stresses.

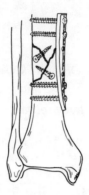

FIGURE 2.8. Neutralization plate.

  2. ***Buttress plate*** — used to protect cortical or cancellous bone from collapsing. It is used to maintain alignment rather than to provide compression. The neutralization plate is used in the shaft of a bone; the buttress plate is used in the metaphyseal region, which is more prone to collapse.

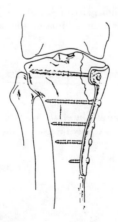

FIGURE 2.9. Buttress plate.

3. ***Dynamic compression plate*** — These plates are self-compressing as a result of oval screw holes with beveled edges and proper screw placement. Fixation screws are placed eccentrically in the screw hole so that they impart a compressive stress to the fracture line as they are tightened.

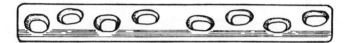

FIGURE 2.10. Dynamic compression plate.

d. ***Cerclage wiring*** — Circumferential wires or bands placed around the bone are used with spiral or oblique fractures.

e. ***Tension band wiring*** — The tension band absorbs the tension and imparts compression to the bone (dynamic compression). By placing tension band wires on the side with maximum tensile stress, the eccentric load is neutralized and compressive stabilization is achieved as well, usually allowing motion at the joint.

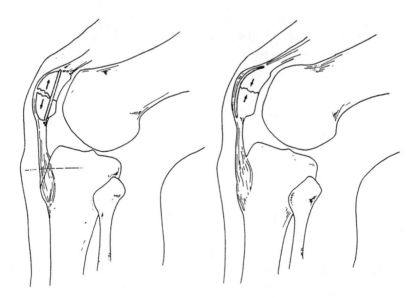

Incorrect: Tensile stress is not neutralized and thus fracture distracts with load.

Correct: Fixation is a site of tensile strength, providing compressive forces at the fracture site.

FIGURE 2.11. Example: Fracture of the patella.

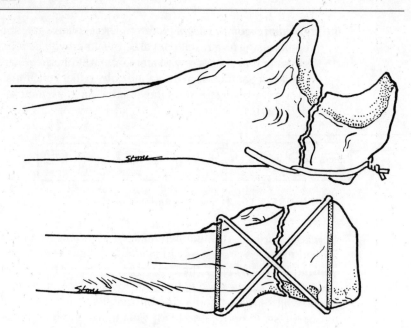

FIGURE 2.12. Example: Transverse fracture of the olecranon.

f. Other means of fixation
  Blade/plate device — This device may be used in both the proximal and distal femur. There are several types.

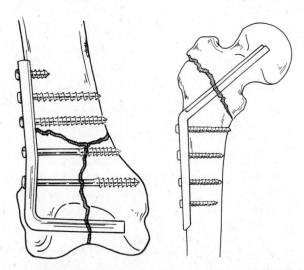

Condylar plate: 95° angle.   Blade plate: 130° angle.

FIGURE 2.13. Blade-type devices.

Intramedullary nail — This device comes in various sizes and is used as a *weight-sharing* rather than a *weight-bearing* device. These provide excellent protection for angular deformity, but are weak in preventing rotation or shortening. They may also be used with transverse screws through the nail to overcome these weaknesses. This type is called an *interlocking IM nail* and may be used as either weight-sharing or weight-bearing, depending on the screw placement.

Semirigid IM nails — These are used with reaming of the intermedullary canal to ensure a contact fit. Flexible IM nails are used without reaming. Multiple small flexible nails may be used.

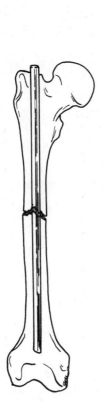 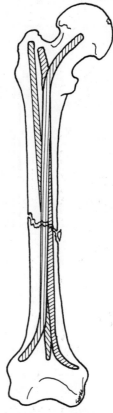

FIGURE 2.14. Semirigid IM nail.

FIGURE 2.15. Flexible rod fixation.

g.   Other internal "fixation"
1.   Bone graft
2.   Suture through soft tissues

EXTERNAL FIXATION DEVICES

External fixation is helpful in cases where rapid stabilization of the fracture is needed or when an open fracture is grossly contaminated. They are also useful in those cases where the remaining bony stock is insufficient to hold internal fixation. These devices are commonly used to manage fractures of the tibia, the pelvic ring, and the distal radius. Screws or pins are inserted percutaneously into the bone above and below the fracture site and attached to one or more rods or bars to form a frame. The connecting bracket may allow great flexibility in changing the alignment of the screws for fine tuning the fracture alignment.

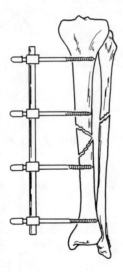

FIGURE 2.16. External fixation of tibial fracture.

COMPLICATIONS OF FRACTURES

Intrinsic complications

- *Infection*
- *Delayed union*
- *Nonunion*
- *Malunion*
- *Avascular necrosis*
- *Shortening*

Extrinsic complications

- *Injury to other tissues*
  Vessels
  Nerves
  Viscera
  Joints
- *Fat embolism*
- *Myositis ossificans*
- *Sudeck's atrophy*
- *Degenerative arthritis*

SOME SPECIAL FEATURES OF FRACTURES IN CHILDREN

Children have very resilient bones and are subject to plastic bowing, greenstick and torus fractures, and other types of incomplete fractures. Fractures through the end of a growing bone may injure the growth plate in various ways. Growth may be delayed, halted, or even accelerated. A classification system was devised by Salter and Harris, which provides a convenient shorthand method for describing these fractures in the radiology report.

The classification is depicted in Figure 2.17.

The abused child: Think of battered child syndrome if multiple bones are fractured without a history of major trauma, especially if there are fractures at different stages of healing. Exuberant callus formation, metaphyseal fractures simulating rickets or infection, or unexplained skull fractures are other tipoffs to the diagnosis.

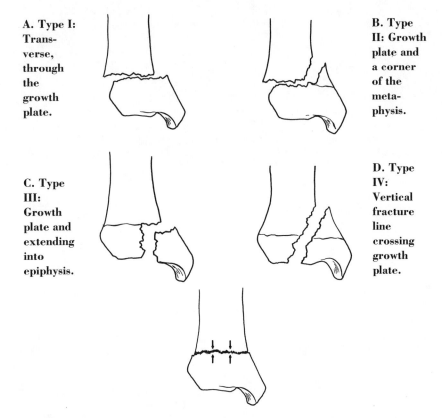

A. Type I: Transverse, through the growth plate.

B. Type II: Growth plate and a corner of the metaphysis.

C. Type III: Growth plate and extending into epiphysis.

D. Type IV: Vertical fracture line crossing growth plate.

E. Type V: "Crush" injury to the growth plate.

FIGURE 2.17. Salter and Harris classification system.

REFERENCES

Richardson, M. L, R. F. Kilcoyne, K. A. Mayo, J. G. Lamont, and W. Hastrup. "Radiographic Evaluation of Modern Orthopedic Fixation Devices," *RadioGraphics* 7:685–701 (1987).

Helms, C. A. *Fundamentals of Skeletal Radiology*. (Philadelphia: W. B. Saunders, 1989).

Rockwood, C. A., Jr. and D. P. Green, Eds. *Fractures in Adults. Fractures in Children*. (Philadelphia: Lippincott, 1984).

Rogers, L. F., Ed. *Radiology of Skeletal Trauma*. (New York: Churchill Livingstone, 1982).

Schultz, R. J., Ed. *The Language of Fractures*. (Huntington, NY: Robert E. Krieger, 1976).

3

TERMINOLOGY FOR JOINT REPLACEMENT IMPLANTS

INTRODUCTION

The introduction of successful joint replacement materials depended on the development of strong, nonallergic metal alloys, slippery plastic surfaces (usually high-density polyethylene), and methylmethacrylate cement as a "grout" to bind the metal stem to the trabecular bone. More recently, prostheses have been devised with a specially formulated surface at the bone interface (porous coating), which allows cementless fixation of the device to the subjacent bone surface.

There are a myriad of orthopedic implants with many brand names for the same basic implant. This chapter provides an overview of implants and common terminology and radiographic appearance.

I.   Hip replacement devices
    A.   Hemiarthroplasty (endoprosthesis)
        1.   Thompson (Figure 3.1)
        2.   Austin Moore
    B   Bipolar
    C.   Total hip replacement
        1.   Charnley (Figure 3.2)
        2.   Triad or DF-80
    D.   Surface replacement
        1.   Tharies (Figure 3.3)

II. Knee replacement
    A.   Total knee (Figure 3.4)
        1.   Polycentric
        2.   Geomedic
        3.   Total condylar
        4.   Posterior stabilizing
        5.   Cruciate sacrificing vs. cruciate retaining
    B.   Hemiarthroplasty
        1.   Marmor (Figure 3.5)
    C.   Patellofemoral replacement

III. Shoulder replacement
    A.   Hemiarthroplasty
        1.   Neer
    B.   Total shoulder
        1.   Neer (Figure 3.6)
        2.   Michael Reese

IV. Small joint arthroplasty (Swanson)
    A.   Hemiarthroplasty
    B.   Double stem (Figure 3.7)

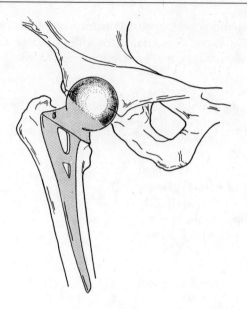

FIGURE 3.1. Thompson endoprosthesis.

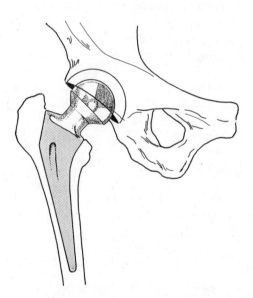

FIGURE 3.2. Charnley prosthesis.

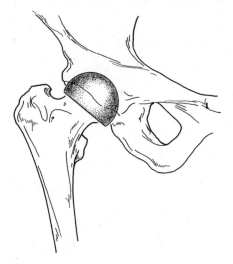

FIGURE 3.3. Tharies surface replacement.

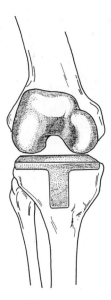

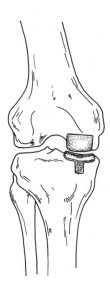

FIGURE 3.4.
Total knee
replacement.

FIGURE 3.5.
Marmor hemi-
arthroplasty.

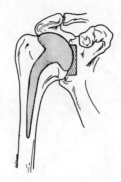

FIGURE 3.6. Neer prosthesis.

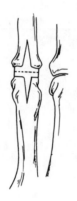

FIGURE 3.7. Swanson prosthesis.

V. Complications of joint prostheses

A number of conditions can develop that cause a prosthesis to fail. These include:

- *Prosthesis loosening*
- *Infection*
- *Dislocation*
- *Malalignment*
- *Instability*
- *Fracture of the prosthesis or of the bone (Figure 3.8)*
- *Cement extrusion*
- *Allergic reaction to the metal or the plastic*
- *Heterotopic bone formation*

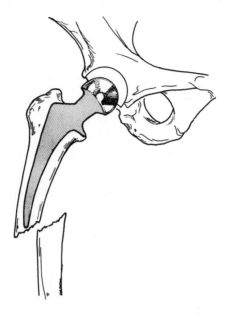

FIGURE 3.8. Fracture of the femur
at the point of maximum stress.

REFERENCES

Rabin, D. N., A. Ali, C. Smith, J. R. Charters, R. A. Kubicka, H. Rabin, and S. Rabin S. "Problem Prostheses: The Radiologic Evaluation of Total Joint Replacement," *RadioGraphics* 7:1107–1127 (1987).

Richardson, M. L., R. F. Kilcoyne, K. A. Mayo, J. G. Lamont, and W. Hastrup. "Radiographic Evaluation of Modern Orthopedic Fixation Devices," *RadioGraphics* 7:685–701 (1987).

4

FRACTURES OF THE SHOULDER AND HUMERUS

ANATOMY OF THE SHOULDER REGION

Diagnosis and management of injuries about the shoulder require an understanding of several soft tissue structures and their relationship to bony injury. Important soft tissues include:

- *Shoulder joint capsule and labrum*
- *Rotator cuff*
- *Tendon of the long head of the biceps*
- *Coracoclavicular ligaments (CC)*
- *Acromioclavicular ligaments (AC)*
- *Coracoacromial ligament (CA)*

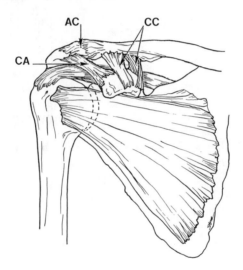

FIGURE 4.1. The acromioclavicular joint.

Injuries to the acromioclavicular joint are divided into six types:

I — Stretching of the acromioclavicular ligaments

II — Disruption of the acromioclavicular ligaments

III — Disruption of the acromio- and coracoclavicular ligaments (or coracoid fracture)

IV — Type III plus superior and posterior displacement of the lateral clavicle

V — Type III plus marked superior displacement of the lateral clavicle

VI — AC ligament disruption with lateral clavicle displaced inferiorly below the acromion or the coracoid

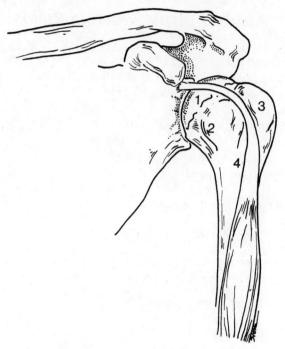

FIGURE 4.2. Segments of the proximal humerus.

The proximal humerus may be divided into four segments:

1. Anatomic neck and articular surface
2. Lesser tuberosity, where the subscapularis tendon attaches
3. Greater tuberosity with the attachment of the supraspinatus and the external rotators
4. Surgical neck and shaft of the humerus

CLASSIFICATION OF HUMERAL FRACTURES

Codman, in a text written in the 1930s, emphasized the importance of displacement of proximal humeral fractures as a cause for poor healing. In 1970, Neer refined the classification and stated that displacement of 1 cm or more, or angulation of more than 45°, meant the fracture was considered significantly displaced. Less displacement was considered *minimal displacement,* regardless of the amount of comminution. The term *fracture-dislocation* means that the articular segment is outside the joint space and is no longer in congruous contact with the glenoid fossa.

The classification scheme that employs the four segment concept depends on which segments are displaced or angulated. In other words, a *three-part fracture* means that all three segments are either displaced by more than 1.0 cm or angulated more than 45°. If there is also a fourth segment that is fractured but not displaced, it is not considered in the classification and does not justify the diagnosis of a *four-part fracture.*

Roentgenographic Exam

An AP in the plane of the glenohumeral joint and an axillary lateral view will usually suffice and can be carried out on most traumatized patients. If pain prevents obtaining an adequate axillary, a transscapular lateral may suffice, or computed tomography (CT) may be necessary to define the extent of the injury. Weight-holding views and the axillary view provide valuable information about the distal end of the clavicle and the acromion. Impingement by a bony spur arising from the anterior acromion and pressing against the supraspinatus tendon can be seen best with an AP view taken with 30° of caudal angulation.

FRACTURES OF THE PROXIMAL HUMERUS

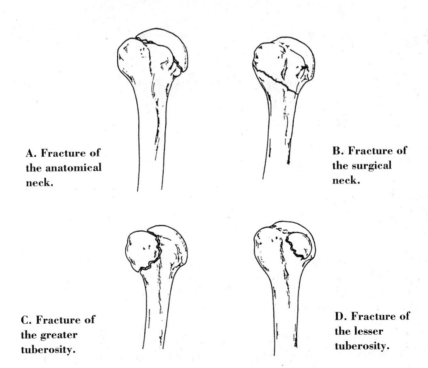

A. Fracture of
the anatomical
neck.

B. Fracture of
the surgical
neck.

C. Fracture of
the greater
tuberosity.

D. Fracture of
the lesser
tuberosity.

FIGURE 4.3. Examples of fractures about the shoulder.

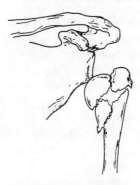

FIGURE 4.3.E. Four-part fracture-disloca-tion.

FRACTURES OF THE CLAVICLE

Fractures of the clavicle usually involve the middle third and are not difficult to diagnose. Fractures of the medial end may extend into the sternoclavicular joint and may be associated with injury to the subclavian artery. CT is helpful in these cases. Fractures of the lateral end of the clavicle are discussed under acromioclavicular (AC) joint injuries.

FRACTURES OF THE SCAPULA

Scapular fractures are divided into

- Neck
- Acromial process
- Spinous process or base of the acromion
- Genoid fossa
- Coracoid process
- Body

Intraarticular fractures of the glenoid may require operative repair. CT is helpful in defining the extent of these fractures.

Associated Injuries
Injuries to the soft tissues about the shoulder can be more significant than the bony damage. With anterior dislocations, there will frequently be an associated tear of the glenoid labrum or anterior glenoid lip fracture

(Bankart lesion). Also with anterior dislocations, an impaction fracture of the posterior humeral head may occur as the head slides over the anterior glenoid labrum and produces a notched defect (Hill-Sachs lesion). With posterior dislocations, analogous "reverse" lesions may occur. Capsular disruption and tears of the rotator cuff often reflect the velocity of the injury. Soft tissue adhesions, restriction of motion, and recurrent dislocations may follow. Neurologic injury may occur, most commonly to the axillary nerve. There is early hypesthesia over the lateral-proximal arm, and later a variable degree of "deltoid paresis". On X-ray this will cause inferior subluxation of the humeral head. This paresis usually resolves in time. Brachial plexus injury is usually seen with high velocity injuries to the neck and upper chest. Vascular injuries may occur, especially in the elderly with vessel wall calcification.

Problems and Complications

Nonunion — This is often the result of interposed soft tissues, muscle pull between the fragments, or distraction due to gravity.

Malunion — This occurs with rotation or displacement of fracture fragments secondary to muscle pull.

Avascular necrosis — This is most commonly seen after four-part fractures that leave the articular segment without the soft tissue attachments and vascular supply of either the greater or lesser tuberosity.

FRACTURES OF THE HUMERAL SHAFT

Two views of the fracture are needed. Both the shoulder and elbow joints should be examined on X-ray.

Classification

The humeral shaft begins just above the insertion of the pectoralis major muscle and extends to the supracondylar ridges below. In addition to the usual terminology for fracture classification, mention of the level of fracture is helpful:

1. Above the pectoralis major insertion
2. Below pectoralis major but above deltoid
3. Below the deltoid insertion

These muscle insertions will influence greatly the subsequent displacement of the fracture fragments.

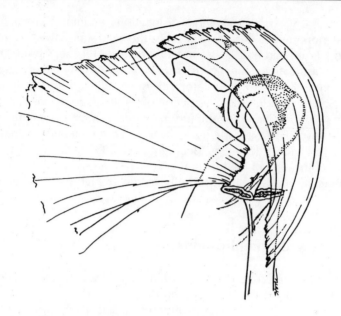

FIGURE 4.4. Fracture below the insertion of the pectoralis
major and above the deltoid.

Associated Injuries

The radial nerve is at risk of injury in fractures of the distal one third, especially spiral-type fractures. Five to ten percent of humeral shaft fractures will have associated damage to the radial nerve. The risk of radial nerve damage is increased by movement of the forearm. This is the main reason that the technologist should never externally rotate the acutely injured humerus when radiographing it. The median and ulnar nerves may also be injured, but much less commonly.

Injuries to the brachial artery are surgical emergencies. Angiography may be required to determine the level of injury.

Treatment and Complications

Indications for internal fixation include segmental fractures, pathologic fractures, low humeral shaft fractures (to protect elbow motion), fractures associated with vascular injury, spiral fractures, and excessive shortening. Delayed union or nonunion is most commonly seen in transverse, midshaft fractures that have minimal bone contact. Interposed soft tissues may be a significant factor. In most series a minimum of 4 months treatment is required before a fracture can be classified as a nonunion. Secondary treatment with rigid internal fixation and bone grafting usually leads to bony union. Another problem is the occurrence of pathologic fractures, because the humerus is a common site of metastatic disease. Internal fixation of these fractures will not interfere with radiotherapy or chemo-therapy.

REFERENCE

Neer, C. "Displaced proximal humeral fractures. Part 1. Classification and Evaluation," *J. Bone Jt. Surg.* 52A: 1077–1089 (1970).

5

FRACTURES AND DISLOCATIONS OF THE ELBOW AND FOREARM

INTRODUCTION

Fractures about the elbow account for approximately 6% of all treated fractures. The combination of complex bony structures and muscle attachments gives this joint very little inherent stability following trauma. Fractures will often cause disruption of interlocking bone surfaces. The muscles that attach to the various fragments and cross the joint line are likely to produce persistent displacement and make reduction difficult.

The elbow joint is complex and a basic understanding of its anatomy is very helpful in describing injuries to this area. It is composed of the humeroulnar, humeroradial, and radioulnar articulations. The axis of the humeroulnar joint determines the arc of elbow flexion/extension. With respect to the body, the forearm moves to a valgus position with elbow extension. The functional significance of the so-called carrying angle is self-evident. It varies from 5° to 20°, with a mean of 15° in adults. Residual deformity of this angle may follow fractures of the elbow and is often described as cubitus varus or cubitus valgus (when compared with the normal contralateral carrying angle).

PERTINENT ANATOMY AND LANDMARKS

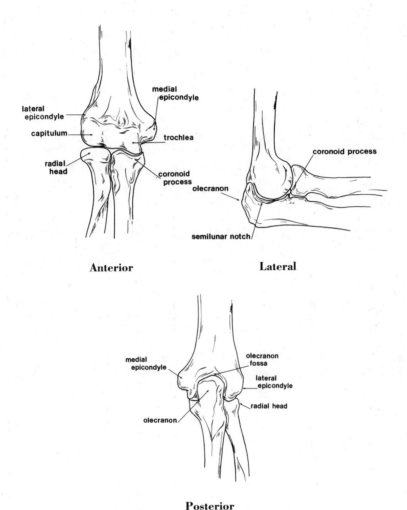

FIGURE 5.1. Anatomy of elbow and forearm.

Important Structures and Attachments

Humerus

1.   Trochlea: the grooved articular surface of the medial condyle of the humerus.

2.   Capitulum: the hemispherical articulating surface of the lateral condyle.
3.   Lateral epicondyle: attachment for the collateral ligament and the superficial extensor muscles of the forearm.
4.   Medial epicondyle: attachment for the collateral ligament and the forearm flexor muscles. The ulnar nerve passes posteriorly.

Ulna

1.   Olecranon: the triceps tendon inserts here.
2.   Semilunar notch: the articulating surface of the ulna. A smooth notch between the olecranon and coronoid processes with a central ridge that fits the corresponding groove of the trochlea.

Radius

1.   Radial head: the concave head articulates with the capitulum of the humerus. The head fits into the radial notch of the ulna and forms a pivot joint. It is surrounded by the strong, densely fibrous anular ligament.

Fat Pads

These so-called Haversian glands lie between the synovial capsule and the more superficial fibrous capsule of the elbow joint. The anterior fat pad is barely visible on the lateral view in normal elbows as a thin, black strip parallel to the humeral shaft. The posterior fat pad is not normally visible and lies deep within the olecranon fossa. Distension of the joint with effusion or hemarthrosis will displace these fat pads and produce the so-called fat pad sign. In trauma, this is evidence of an occult, often intraarticular, fracture (usually of the radial head).

FRACTURES OF THE DISTAL HUMERUS

Fractures of the distal humerus are common in children. Because of the various ossification centers present and the attachment of important forearm flexor muscles, it is important not to underestimate the severity of the injury.

In children 58% of elbow injuries are supracondylar fractures, 13% involve the lateral condyle, and 10% involve the medial condyle of the distal humerus. Angulation or rotatory displacement of supracondylar fractures in children is difficult to assess in plaster with the elbow in the flexed position. Failure to recognize malalignment will lead to permanent deformity.

Extension-type Supracondylar Fracture

Extraarticular fractures occur through the medial and lateral columns of the distal humerus. Extension-type fractures occur from a fall on the outstretched arm with the elbow in extension. The distal fragment is displaced posterior to the shaft of the humerus. It may also show lateral or medial displacement. These fractures are more common in children, presumably because the anterior capsule and the collateral ligaments are stronger than bone.

These fractures are inherently unstable and are difficult to reduce. Close scrutiny will often reveal axial rotation of the distal fragment and/ or angulation in the medial-lateral plane. This must all be taken into consideration in assessing reduction.

Guidelines For Adequate Reduction:

There should be nearly 100% apposition of fracture surfaces.

There should be no rotational malalignment between the proximal and distal fragments.

Condylar angulation (anteriorly) should be within 20° of the normal condyle-shaft angle.

In children, Bauman's angle of the distal humerus on the AP view should be 70°.

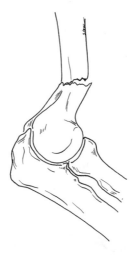

FIGURE 5.2. Extension type of supracondylar fracture.

Treatment

Usually closed reduction is attempted first. Radiographic confirmation of anatomic alignment is mandatory. Oblique views and films of the opposite elbow will often help to assess reduction. Once reduction is achieved, flexion of the elbow will help to stabilize the fracture. However, flexion may further impair circulation if there is a great deal of swelling. Due to the unstable nature of these fractures, follow-up X-rays should be obtained frequently in the first and second weeks to make certain that reduction has been maintained.

If closed reduction is unsuccessful, internal stabilization is often needed. A fracture of the forearm in the same limb ("floating elbow") is considered an indication for internal stabilization. The types of internal fixation include percutaneous K wires, often used in children, and various plate/screw combinations, more frequently seen in adults.

Flexion-type Supracondylar Fracture

This is caused by a fall or blow against the posterior aspect of the flexed elbow. It is characterized by anterior displacement of the distal fragment. It is a relatively rare injury (~2% of supracondylar fractures), but it is more likely to be open because of the direct trauma. X-rays will usually show a fracture line on lateral films that slopes from proximal anteriorly to distal posteriorly. This will appear transverse on the AP views.

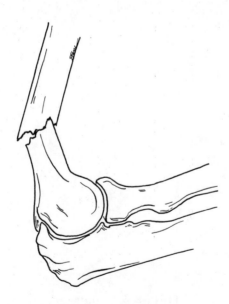

FIGURE 5.3. Flexion fracture.

Treatment

Reduction requires manipulation different from the extension fracture, and stability of the flexion fracture is enhanced by extension of the elbow, taking advantage of the intact anterior periosteum. Following reduction, factors similar to those discussed under extension injuries apply.

Complications

- **Vascular injuries** — The primary concern is damage to the brachial artery, either as a result of the original injury or at the time of attempted reduction.
- **Volkmann's contracture** — This is now appreciated as the late result of an acute compartment syndrome. Once diagnosed, urgent fasciotomy is indicated.
- **Neurologic injury** — This is reported to occur in ~15% of supracondylar fractures. Usually the injury is a neuropraxia that will gradually resolve. Occasionally a bone fragment will impinge directly upon a nerve. The median and radial nerve are involved with equal frequency; the ulnar is the least likely. Tardy ulnar nerve palsy may develop after childhood fractures. If the fracture heals in an angulated position, the ulnar nerve may be stretched as the upper limb grows in length.
- **Nonunion** — Almost never a problem.
- **Malunion** — It is difficult to assess varus-valgus angulation unless the elbow is extended. Therefore, this deformity may go unrecognized during early treatment. The most common residual deformity is known as a *gunstock deformity* or cubitus varus, which results in functional and cosmetic disability.
- **Loss of rotation** — This may occur commonly in adults after immobilization for any elbow injury. Some authors suggest internal stabilization and early motion to avoid this.
- **Epiphyseal malunion** — Injury to the growth cartilage in children may lead to abnormal angulation with subsequent maturation. Arthrography or tomography may be needed to assess the extent of epiphyseal plate injuries.

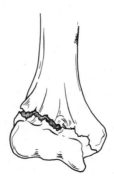

FIGURE 5.4. Transcondylar fracture.

Medial Condylar Fracture

This will have intraarticular extension. It is rare as an isolated injury and may be associated with elbow dislocation. For treatment, closed reduction is attempted. Displacement greater than 2 mm involving the articular surface usually requires open reduction and internal fixation with pins or screws. Intraarticular extension may be difficult to detect in children, in which case an elbow arthrogram is helpful.

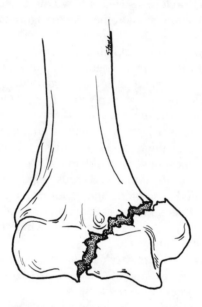

FIGURE 5.5. Medial condylar fracture.

Complications

- *Posttraumatic arthritis*
- *Damage to the epiphyseal plate in children with late deformity*
- *Injury to the ulnar nerve*
- *Loss of elbow motion*

Medial Epicondylar Fracture

This is usually an avulsion fracture and may be associated with elbow dislocation. Although the fracture is extraarticular, the fragment may become trapped within the joint. In treatment, 10 mm of displacement is acceptable. If more than that, or if the elbow is unstable, repair or pinning may be required.

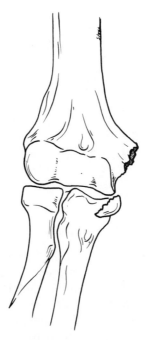

FIGURE 5.6. Medial epicondylar fracture.

Complications

- *Unrecognized intraarticular fragment*
- *Injury to the ulnar nerve*
- *Elbow instability: The medial collateral ligament attaches to the medial epicondyle and is a major stabilizer of the elbow joint.*

Lateral Condylar Fracture

These often have intraarticular extension and may fracture through the capitulum or at its base, leaving behind an avascular fragment. If the fragment is not stabilized, the amount of displacement may increase with time because of the pull of the extensor muscles.

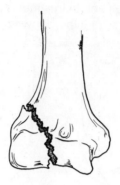

**FIGURE 5.7. Lateral
condylar fracture.**

Treatment

If displaced, this fracture requires open reduction and internal fixation.

Complications

Inaccurate reduction, or loss of reduction, leads to valgus collapse, posttraumatic arthritis, and late ulnar nerve palsy. In children, this is a Salter-Harris IV type of fracture and may therefore damage the epiphyseal plate. This may lead to growth arrest or overgrowth of the lateral epiphysis. Either of these may cause late deformity, and follow-up X-rays at 3, 6, 9 and 12 months are usually recommended.

Intercondylar Y or T Fracture

These usually involve high-velocity trauma with significant intraarticular injury. Frequently X-rays will underestimate the degree of intraarticular comminution.

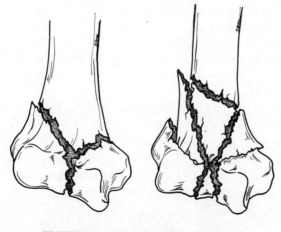

A. Simple
Y fracture.

B. Comminuted intercondylar fracture.

FIGURE 5.8. Intercondylar fracture.

Treatment

If the fragments are large enough, open reduction and stable rigid fixation with early motion give the best results. Interfragmentary screws and neutralization/buttress plates are usually used. It is important to reestablish the trochlear joint surface and condylar width as closely as possible. If the fracture is very comminuted, then olecranon pin traction may be needed.

Complications

These may be open fractures with soft tissue injury. There is increased risk of nerve or vessel injury with this fracture pattern. Loss of motion after healing may be a serious problem, especially if early motion with treatment cannot be instituted. Posttraumatic arthritis is common.

Osteochondral Fracture

These may occur with elbow dislocation and are difficult or impossible to demonstrate with plain films and may require air arthrotomography or computed tomography.

Complications

These fragments may cause symptoms of internal derangement in the elbow joint and may lead to posttraumatic arthritis.

FRACTURES OF THE PROXIMAL RADIUS

The most commonly injured area in the elbow is the radial head. The articulations and soft tissue attachments of the proximal radius and ulna are complex. A basic understanding of anatomy is necessary in order to diagnose bony injury.

Radial Head Fracture

The mechanism of fracture may be direct trauma or indirect axial loading through the radial shaft. The radial head does not fully contact the capitulum until the elbow flexes to 135°. However, it is in constant contact with the lesser sigmoid notch of the ulna. The significance of this is that small fractures will affect forearm supination/pronation to a much greater extent than elbow flexion/extension.

The classification is best made by a careful description of the location and extent of the fracture, the amount of displacement, and the amount of the radial head that is involved.

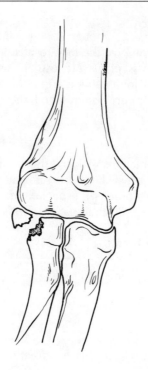

FIGURE 5.9. **Radial head fracture.**

Mason classification of radial head fractures:

I — Undisplaced fracture
II — Marginal fracture with variable size and displacement
III — Comminuted fracture with total head involvement
IV — Fracture associated with elbow dislocation (plus severe soft tissue injury)

Occult fractures are common and almost always are associated with an effusion (as manifest by a positive fat pad sign). There may be associated fracture of the capitulum.

Radial Neck Fracture
The mechanism of fracture is the same as radial head fracture. The most common type is impacted, but marked angulation can occur.

Fractures of the Proximal Radial Shaft
The biceps and supinator muscles are both supinators of the forearm and insert on the proximal radius. Fractures distal to the area of biceps attachment will tend to have the proximal fragment supinated with respect to the distal fragment.

FRACTURES OF THE ULNA

Fractures of the Olecranon and Coronoid Processes

Fractures of the olecranon process usually result from a direct blow or indirect avulsion from pull of the triceps brachii. Ulnar nerve injuries may accompany these fractures. A true lateral radiograph is important for evaluating alignment.

Fractures of the coronoid process are often seen with posterior dislocations of the elbow.

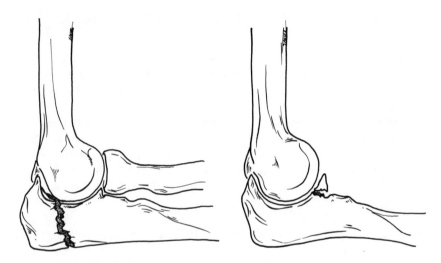

A. Fracture of the olecranon process.   **B. Fracture of the coronoid process.**

FIGURE 5.10.

DISLOCATIONS OF THE ELBOW

Isolated radial head dislocations occur much more commonly in children. The combination of radial head dislocation with fracture of the ulnar shaft is known as Monteggia fracture-dislocation. Isolated ulnar dislocation is usually in a posterior direction.

Fractures that are commonly associated with elbow dislocations include

* *Avulsion of the medial or lateral epicondyle*
* *Avulsion of the coronoid process*
* *Fracture of the radial head or neck*
* *Fracture of the capitulum*

Complications

- *Restricted motion*
- *Unrecognized fractures*
- *Intraarticular fragments*
- *Heterotopic ossification or myositis ossificans*
- *Ulnar nerve injury*
- *Brachial artery injury*

Fractures of the Radial and Ulnar Shafts

Most of these are produced by direct trauma. In adults they are usually treated by open reduction and internal fixation. Malalignment and malrotation are common complications and lead to limitation of supination and pronation.

Because of the complex articulations and soft tissue attachments of the radius and ulna, injury to one bone by a blow has an effect on the other bone. If a fracture of the radius or ulna is seen on X-ray and there is shortening then there should be

- *Fracture of the other forearm bone, or*
- *Disruption of the proximal radioulnar joint (Monteggia fracture), or*
- *Disruption of the distal radioulnar joint (Galeazzi fracture).*

Malrotation is a difficult problem to correct in the treatment of these fractures, and, therefore, internal fixation is frequently utilized in adults.

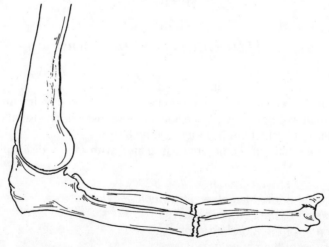

FIGURE 5.11. Fractures of the radial and ulnar shafts.

REFERENCES

Fahey, J. J. "Fractures of the Elbow in Children," *A.A.O.S. Instructional Course Lectures, Vol. 17* (St. Louis, MO: C.V. Mosby, 1960), pp. 13-46.

Hansen, P. E., D. A. Barnes, and H. S. Tulles. "Arthrographic diagnosis of injury pattern in the distal humerus of an infant," *J. Pediatr. Ortho.* 2:569–572 (1982).

Noren, H. G. "Roentgenologic visualization of the extracapsular fat. Its importance in the diagnosis of traumatic injuries to the elbow," *Acta Radiol.* 42:205–210 (1954).

6

INJURIES TO THE WRIST AND HAND

THE DISTAL RADIUS AND ULNA

Fractures of the distal radius and ulna are quite common from a fall on the outstretched hand. In 1814 Abraham Colles published an excellent description of the distal radial fracture with volar angulation and dorsal displacement, noting its frequent occurrence in older persons.

The distal radius has a broad concave articular surface that angles approximately 11° volarly and 25° ulnarly. This angle is disrupted in serious injuries. Minor injuries may tear supporting ligaments. More serious injuries may tear the triangular fibrocartilage between the distal ulna and the carpus. Dislocations of the radial-carpal and radial-ulnar joints are usually reduced with supination.

If the injury causes a discrepancy in the length between the radius and ulna, pain and symptoms of derangement of the distal radial-ulnar joint can result. Treatment of this disabling condition may include repair of the triangular cartilage, repair of the distal radial-ulnar joint, and excision of the distal ulna (Darrach procedure).

Wrist Fracture Classification (Palmer, 1983)

I. Fracture pattern
    Incomplete ("buckle" or "torus" fracture)
    Impacted
    Transverse
    Oblique
    Comminuted

II. Fracture extent
    Styloid fracture
    Extraarticular
    Intraarticular

III. Angulation
    Volar
    Dorsal

IV. Displacement
    Dorsal
    Volar
    Proximal (shortening)
    Radial
    Unar

64

V.   Ulnar injury
       Styloid fracture
       Disrupted radioulnar joint
       Ulnar complex injury (distal ulna and triangular fibrocartilage)

The radiographic report should take all of the above factors into account. Regarding angulation of distal radial fractures, there is a confusing terminology regarding angulation due to a failure to specify whether the description refers to the fracture itself or to the position of the distal fragment. Strictly speaking, a description of the fracture would state volar angulation if the apex of the fracture is volar. However, it is common practice to describe angulation of distal radial fractures with reference to the position of the distal fragment rather than the fracture itself. The radiologist should always indicate whether he or she is referring to "dorsal displacement of the distal fragment" or "apex volar angulation at the fracture site".

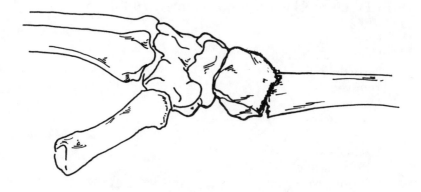

FIGURE 6.1. Angulation of typical Colles fracture.

THE CARPAL BONES

The carpal joints are formed by eight bones linked by multiple ligaments. The most common serious injury in the carpal region is fracture of the scaphoid. This injury, as well as other fractures and dislocations, may be accompanied by significant ligamentous injuries and instability. So-called dorsal chip fractures may indicate ligamentous injury (Dobyns, 1980).

The complete radiographic evaluation of the wrist may require additional views with ulnar and radial deviation, flexion and extension, or stress.

Classification of Carpal Injuries
- *Scaphoid fractures*
- *Lunate or perilunate dislocations*
- *Posttraumatic carpal instability*

The items in the above classification are not mutually exclusive. Frequently there is association between the various injuries, such that dislocations may be associated with fractures and instability results from ligamentous tears.

Fractures of the scaphoid may be difficult to diagnose and there may be problems in healing. Complications include malunion with rotation of the distal fragment, nonunion, avascular necrosis of the proximal pole, and associated ligamentous injuries.

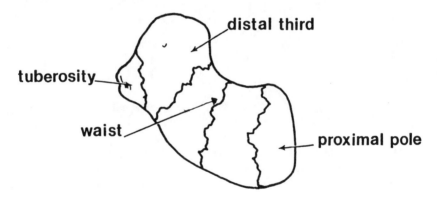

FIGURE 6.2.   Types of scaphoid fractures.

Injuries to the Greater and Lesser Carpal Arcs
Lesser arc injuries (Figure 6.3) occur in the following patterns with progressively increasing injury:

1. Scapholunate dissociation or rotatory subluxation of the scaphoid
2. Dislocation of the capitate or perilunate dislocation
3. Midcarpal dislocation or disruption of the triquetrolunate articulation
4. Complete lunate disruption

Greater arc injuries (Figure 6.3) require fracture of the scaphoid, capitate, hamate and/or triquetrum, usually associated with a dislocation. The most common greater arc injury is a fracture through the waist of the scaphoid with perilunate instability (Yeager and Dalinka, 1985).

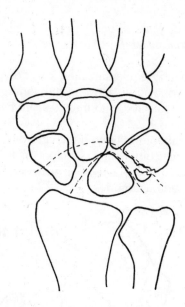

FIGURE 6.3. The greater and lesser arcs of the carpus.

Classification of Posttraumatic Carpal Instability

Ligament injuries, with or without fracture, may lead to an unstable wrist. The scaphoid forms the radial link between the proximal and distal carpal rows and is frequently fractured with ligament injuries. Ligamentous instability usually alters the relationship of the lunate to the other wrist bones.

1. ***Dorsal intercalated segment instability (DISI)*** — The distal surface of the lunate tilts dorsally. The scaphoid usually tilts volarly, increasing the angle between the two bones. The space between the scaphoid and lunate is usually widened.
2. ***Volar intercalated segment instability (VISI)*** — The lunate tilts volarly and the distal capitate tilts dorsally, increasing the capitolunate angle. This VISI pattern may be a normal variant in persons with lax ligaments (Yeager and Dalinka, 1985).

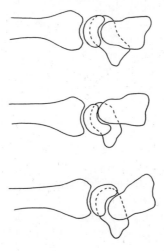

FIGURE 6.4. The scapholunate relationship on lateral radiographs.

METACARPAL FRACTURES

Classification by Anatomic Area

Fracture of the Metacarpal Head

This usually occurs from a crushing or penetrating injury; it frequently is comminuted. The fracture is distal to the collateral ligament/capsule attachment and has very little stability or soft tissue support to aid reduction.

A radiographic view made in the AP projection with the MCP joints flexed and the tube angled 15° ulnarly is helpful in evaluating metacarpal head fractures (Lane, 1977).

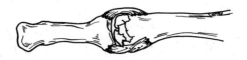

FIGURE 6.5. Fracture of the metacarpal head.

Fracture of the Metacarpal Neck

This is frequently unstable because of comminution of the volar cortex. These fractures tend to return to the original angulation after reduction.

The lateral view is important, because each metacarpal is a different length, and the metacarpal head can be used as a reference point to trace cortical lines and to assess fractures. This is the only view that will accurately show angular deformity in the sagittal plane. It is also important for the assessment of the metacarpal-phalangeal and carpometacarpal relationships.

The most common fracture is of the fifth metacarpal neck with apex dorsal angulation (boxer's fracture). Up to 40° of dorsal angulation can be accepted and still give satisfactory results.

By contrast, fractures of the second and third metacarpals require near perfect reduction because there is very little carpometacarpal compensatory motion, and slight distal deformity can lead to large functional loss.

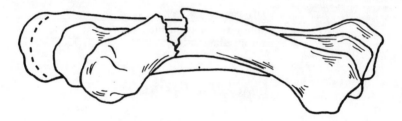

FIGURE 6.6. Fracture of the fifth metacarpal.

Treatment — Following reduction most of these fractures are managed in a cast. Some favor percutaneous pinning, others use plates and screws, and for very comminuted fractures it may be necessary to use some means of external fixation to maintain length and alignment.

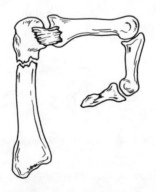

FIGURE 6.7. Reduction of metacarpal neck fracture.

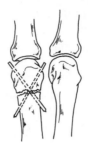

**FIGURE 6.8.   Crossed K wires
used as transfixation pins.**

Dislocations of the Metacarpal-Carpal Joints

These may occur with or without fracture and may be intra- or extraarticular. Diagnosis may be difficult unless the carpal-metacarpal articulations are carefully studied in both lateral and oblique projections. Reduction of dislocations at the base of the fourth or fifth metacarpal may be difficult because of the pull of the extensor carpi ulnaris on the metacarpal shaft.

Fracture of the Thumb Metacarpal

The first metacarpal has a complex articulation with the trapezium to allow apposition and grasp. Most fractures involve the base of the first metacarpal. There are four types described, and management and prognosis depend on whether the fracture is intraarticular or not.

Intraarticular fracture-dislocation (Bennett's fracture) — The shaft is avulsed from the volar fragment, which is held by the strong anterior ligament. The shaft fracture is displaced by the pull of the adductor pollicis and the abductor pollicis longus. Treatment frequently requires internal fixation with K wires for stabilization.

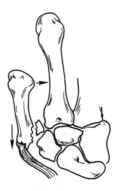

**FIGURE 6.9.
Bennet's fracture.**

Comminuted intraarticular fracture (Rolando's fracture) — This is the least common type. Treatment is difficult because of frequent inability to reduce the comminuted fragments, and posttraumatic arthritis is common.

Extraarticular fractures — This is the most common type. The prognosis is good, even if there is some residual angulation.

Growth plate injuries in children (Salter-Harris II) — These are usually easily reduced and have a good prognosis.

Metacarpal-Phalangeal Joint Dislocation

The phalanx is subluxed or dislocated dorsally. If the volar plate is disrupted, closed reduction will be impossible because the plate becomes lodged between the metacarpal head and the proximal phalanx. This injury may present with less deformity than the simple dislocation without volar plate impingement. Therefore, the diagnosis may be missed.

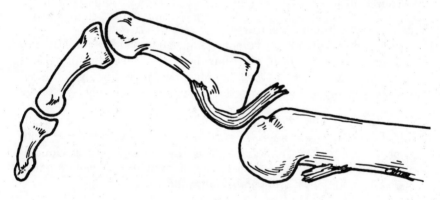

FIGURE 6.10. Metacarpal-phalangeal joint dislocation.

Phalangeal Fractures

Proximal Phalangeal Shaft Fractures

These fractures are frequently nondisplaced and thus are stable. Spiral fractures may rotate and/or shorten. Unstable fractures frequently present with volar angulation as a result of tendon attachments and pull.

Clinical exam and comparison with the "normal" hand are very important for estimating rotational deformity. Radiographs are not accurate in measuring rotation. The fingers should move together with flexion without overriding and should point toward the scaphoid tubercle.

Intraarticular Fractures

Nondisplaced Fractures
The lack of displacement must be confirmed by X-rays in multiple planes. If there is less than 1 mm displacement, then most surgeons recommend treatment with protected early range of motion (i.e., "buddy taping"). The prognosis is good.

Fracture of the Condyle
This fracture is frequently displaced and always involves a significant portion of the articular surface. Chondral fractures may exist and may not be apparent on plain X-ray. An arthrogram of the joint may help in showing these fragments. Treatment is usually reduction into anatomic position and pin fixation for stability. Intraarticular incongruity in displaced fractures may lead to deformity and malalignment of the finger.

Avulsion Fractures
These injuries almost always reflect disruption of a collateral ligament and thus there is the possibility of joint instability. Treatment is usually splinting or immobilization for a brief time if the fracture is small and nondisplaced, followed by protected motion. If the fragment is sizable and displaced, then it is usually reduced and pinned.

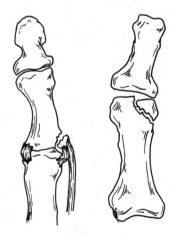

FIGURE 6.11.
Fracture of the proximal phalanx of the thumb.

FIGURE 6.12.
Fracture of the proximal phalangeal condyle.

Fractures of the Middle Phalanx
This is the least commonly fractured of the phalanges. The insertions of the central slip of the extensor tendon and of the flexor sublimis are important deforming factors.

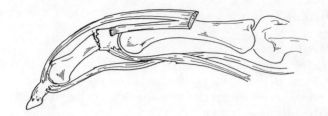

FIGURE 6.13. Fracture at the base of the middle phalanx.

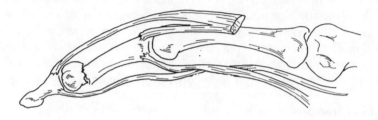

FIGURE 6.14. Fracture at the neck of the middle phalanx.

Dorsal and Volar Lip Fractures

If these are not displaced more than 1 mm, simple protected motion usually leads to good results. If displaced, these fractures reflect PIP joint disruption and are often associated with subluxation or dislocation.

Dorsal lip fractures may indicate disruption of the central slip of the extensor hood and may be associated with a boutonniere deformity (flexion of the PIP joint and hyperextension of the DIP joint.) Treatment is usually closed reduction followed by extension splinting.

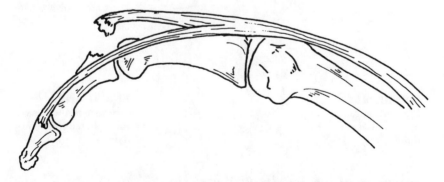

FIGURE 6.15. Boutonniere deformity with dorsal lip avulsion fracture.

Volar lip avulsion is usually treated by closed reduction and splinting in flexion at the PIP joint, but it may require open reduction and internal fixation to maintain joint stability because of the important soft tissue attachments (volar plate and collateral ligaments). Without fixation, the middle phalangeal shaft may subluxe dorsally with resultant joint incongruity.

Complications include stiffness, malunion from rotation, angulation or shortening, and nonunion.

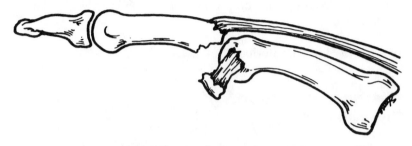

FIGURE 6.16. Volar lip avulsion.

Fractures of the Distal Phalanx

These represent greater than 50% of all hand fractures. The distal phalanx of the long finger is most commonly involved.

Avulsion Injuries

Mallet finger

This is a term that refers to a deformity of a flexed DIP joint following disruption of the extensor tendon continuity (also known as "baseball finger" or "drop finger"). This deformity is associated with three degrees of injury.

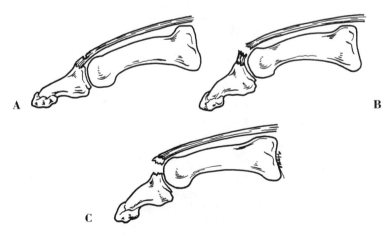

FIGURE 6.17. Mallet finger. A. Partial tear of tendon (5–20° loss). B. Complete tear of tendon (40–45° loss). C. Avulsion of small bony fragment.

Treatment and complications. — Most authors recommend splinting the DIP in extension with some form of external support for 6–10 weeks. K-wire fixation of the DIP joint is also used occasionally. Fixation of the PIP joint (to protect repair) is controversial. When the fracture is intraarticular there is an increased risk of posttraumatic DJD. The dorsal lip fragment is easily disrupted with fixation wires. There is almost always some loss of DIP motion.

Avulsion of Flexor Digitorium Profundus
This is relatively uncommon and is easily missed. The ring finger is the most common site.

Classification (Leddy et al., 1977)

1. Tendon avulsed at attachment site. Retracts into palm
2. Tendon avulsed at attachment and retracts to level of PIP joint (occasionally with fleck of bone)
3. Tendon avulsed with a bony fragment and trapped at distal "pulley" of tendon sheath

Crush Injuries
These injuries may damage the nail bed which can lead to later complications of an epidermoid inclusion cyst or osteomyelitis. Angulated fractures should be reduced and may require pinning.

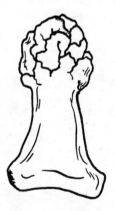

FIGURE 6.18.
"Crushed egg shell":
severe soft tissue
damage.

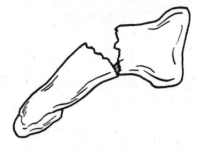

FIGURE 6.19. Transverse: may involve the nail bed and may show significant angulation.

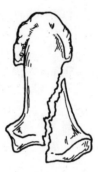

FIGURE 6.20. Longitudinal: relatively stable and rarely displaced.

Treatment

Primarily treatment is to protect soft tissues, with splinting to relieve pain. Transverse, angulated fractures may require reduction and a K-wire fixation pin.

Special Considerations/Complications

Nail bed injuries, inclusion cysts, osteomyelitis, and joint stiffness are all potential sequelae of distal phalangeal fractures.

PIP and DIP stiffness: DIP stiffness may be unavoidable, but stiffness of the PIP joint can be minimized by early motion.

REFERENCES

Dobyns, J. H. and R. L. Lincsheid. "Carpal bone injuries," *Clin. Orthoped.* 149:2-3 (1980).

Lane, C. "Detecting occult fractures of the metacarpal head: The Brewerton view," *J. Hand Surg.* 2:131 (1977).

Leddy, J. P. and J. W. Packer. "Avulsion of the profundus insertion in athletes," *J. Hand Surg.* 2:66-69 (1977).

Mayfield, J. K., R. P. Johnson, and R. F. Kilcoyne. "Carpal dislocations: Pathomechanics and progressive perilunar instability," *J. Hand Surg.* 5:226–241 (1980).

Palmer, A. K., Ed. "Symposium: Distal ulnar injuries," *Contemp. Orthop.* 7:81 (1983).

Yeager, B. A. and M. K. Dalinka. "Radiology of trauma to the wrist: Dislocations, fracture dislocations, and instability patterns," *Skeletal Radiol.* 13:120–130 (1985).

7

PELVIS AND HIP

ACETABULAR FRACTURES

The acetabular hip socket is composed of anterior and posterior rims (lips) and columns, a roof or dome, a thin medial section called the *quadrilateral surface,* and a thicker inferomedial wall called the *teardrop,* because of its appearance on X-ray.

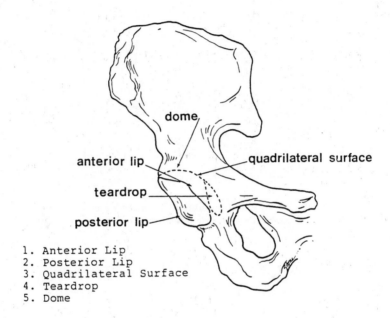

1. Anterior Lip
2. Posterior Lip
3. Quadrilateral Surface
4. Teardrop
5. Dome

FIGURE 7.1. Radiographic components of the acetabular socket.

The radiographic evaluation of the fractured acetabulum should include four views: AP of pelvis, AP centered on affected hip, and right and left obliques of the pelvis to display the anterior and posterior columns of the acetabulum.

The Anterior and Posterior Pelvic Columns

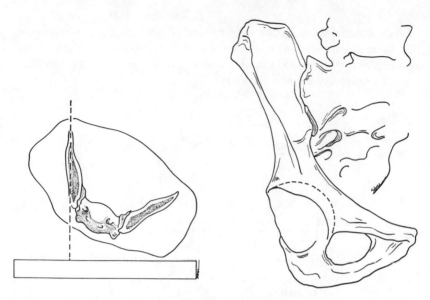

FIGURE 7.2. Anterior column (iliopubic): The anterior iliac crest extending along the anterior ilium to the superior pubic ramus and symphysis.

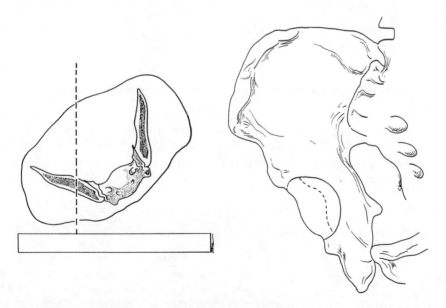

FIGURE 7.3. Posterior column (ilioischial): The ilium from the angle of the sciatic notch caudally to the ischium and ischial tuberosity.

Acetabular Fracture Classification

1. Fracture of posterior rim
2. Fracture of posterior column
3. Fracture of anterior rim
4. Fracture of anterior column
5. Transverse fracture

Most fractures are combinations of these basic patterns.

Specific Fracture Patterns

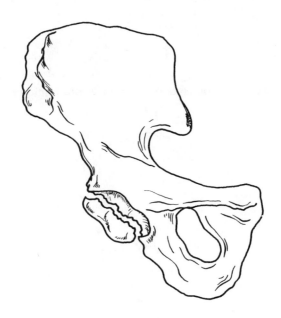

FIGURE 7.4. Posterior rim fracture.

1. This fracture separates a segment of the posterior articular surface, but leaves the major posterior column intact.
2. It is frequently associated with a posterior dislocation of the hip.
3. It may also be associated with impaction of the inner part of the posterior acetabular surface or with femoral head fractures.

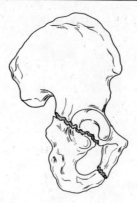

FIGURE 7.5.   Posterior column fractures.

1.   These are usually caused by impaction of the femoral head into the acetabulum, detaching the posterior ilium and ischium.
2.   These may be associated with posterior rim fractures.

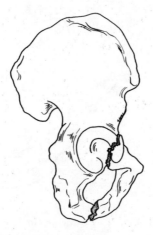

FIGURE 7.6. Anterior column or rim fractures.

1.   Anterior fractures (rim or column) result from separation of the anterior articular lip.
2.   Anterior column fractures disrupt the iliopectineal line.
3.   The fragments may be split either lengthwise or transversely and may carry with them an inner part of the acetabular roof.

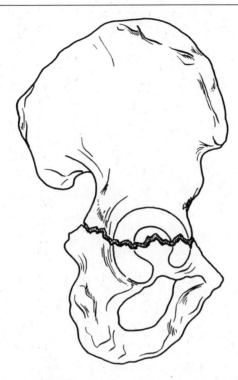

FIGURE 7.7. Transverse fractures.

1. These split the innominate bone through the acetabulum into an upper iliac segment and a lower ischiopubic segment.
2. Both anterior and posterior columns are divided into a superior and inferior segment.
3. They are frequently severely comminuted.

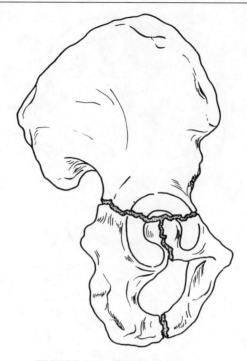

FIGURE 7.8. T-shaped fracture.

Associated or combination fractures

1. T-shaped fractures. This is a combination of a transverse fracture with a vertical split dividing the ischiopubic ramus or extending obliquely through the ischium.
2. Posterior column and posterior rim fractures. Disruption of the posterior column with impaction of the posterior rim, which may create several fragments. Frequently associated with posterior dislocation of the femoral head (which may also disrupt the acetabular roof or "dome").
3. Transverse and posterior rim fractures. Fairly common pattern with femoral head frequently dislocated posteriorly.
4. Anterior rim and posterior column fractures. Femoral head displaced medially with anterior column intact.
5. Fractures of both columns. Complicated acetabular fractures with the posterior element similar to simple posterior column fracture,

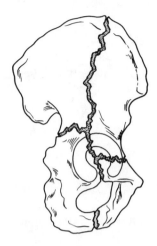

**FIGURE 7.9. Fractures of
both columns.**

and the anterior element variable, usually extending either adjacent
to the acetabular roof or angling upward at the acetabular roof. The
whole articular surface is detached in several pieces and the femoral
head penetrates centrally.

In both column fractures with disruption of the acetabular articular
surface the medial quadrilateral wall and acetabular roof fragments may
be better seen with CT. This can also be valuable for demonstrating
intraarticular fragments that may not be apparent on plain films.

CLASSIFICATION OF PELVIC RING FRACTURES

Pelvic ring fractures, i.e., those involving the anterior and posterior arcs
of the pelvis, can be considered separately from acetabular fractures. The
mechanism of injury is frequently different and aids in the classification
of these injuries. CT is helpful in defining the full extent of the injury,
especially in the region of the sacrum and the sacroiliac joints.

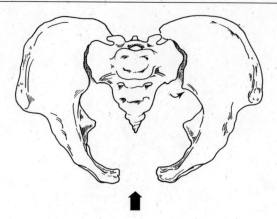

FIGURE 7.10. AP compression.

AP Compression

A direct AP force causes fractures of the pubic ramus, frequently with diastasis. The pubic rami fractures are oriented vertically, which differentiates them from the lateral compression injuries. The anterior sacroiliac ligaments may be torn, giving an "open book" appearance to the pelvis.

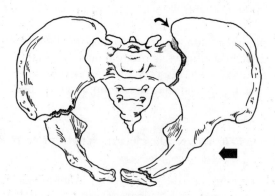

FIGURE 7.11. Lateral compression fracture.

Lateral Compression

This injury results in fractures of the pubic rami, the sacrum and, occasionally, the iliac wing. Since the injury is due to compression, there may not be ligamentous injury. The pubic rami fractures are horizontal or coronal.

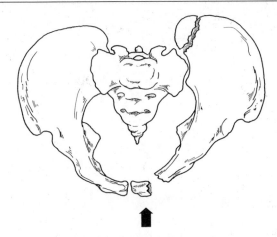

FIGURE 7.12. Vertical shear fracture.

Vertical Shear Fractures (Malgaigne Fractures)

These injuries are caused by a severe vertical force striking lateral to the midline of the pelvis. They generally occur in patients who have fallen or jumped from a height. This type of injury is associated with severe ligamentous disruption and pelvic instability. The fractures not only extend from front to back, but are also directed inferiorly to superiorly.

Complex Pattern

As in most cases of injury, various combinations of fractures occur when the forces are exerted from several directions. Incidentally, the so-called straddle fracture probably does not exist, since most anterior injuries have a posterior component (Young et al., 1986).

INTERNAL FIXATION OF HIP FRACTURES

The principles of internal fixation of hip fractures include restoration of as near an anatomic position as possible and stability of the fracture fragments. Stability should be achieved by reduction and then ensured by fixation.

Devices for Internal Fixation

Many devices are designed to allow impaction with early weight bearing.

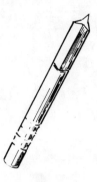

FIGURE 7.13.
Use of tri-flanged
nail.

Tri-Flanged Nail

Useful for intracapsular fractures only. Problems with its use include poor fixation in osteoporotic bone, poor impaction capabilities, and no fixation to the shaft.

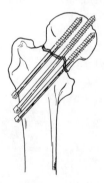

FIGURE 7.14.
Use of multiple
pins.

Multiple Pins

Multiple pins, such as Knowles pins, Hagie pins, and Steinmann pins, are only used for intracapsular fractures. Problems with their use:

- *May penetrate into hip joint or acetabulum (as shown below)*
- *Pinholes are stress risers in the lateral cortex*
- *Difficult to achieve compression at the fracture site*

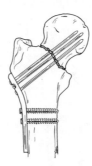

FIGURE 7.15.
Use of multiple
pins with side
plate.

Multiple Pins with Side Plate (Deyerle Apparatus)
Problems with their use:

- *Difficult to use*
- *Femoral shaft may fracture below side plate due to "stress riser" effect*
- *High incidence of osteonecrosis of the femoral head*

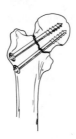

FIGURE 7.16.
Use of multiple
screws.

Multiple Screws
Problems with their use:

- *Technically more difficult: screw threads must not straddle the fracture site or compression effect is lost*
- *Screws should be placed parallel to one another in both planes*
- *If placed too low, the screwhole in the cortex may act as a stress riser and predispose to fracture through the screw hole*

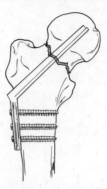

FIGURE 7.17.
Use of nail and side plate combinations.

Nail and Side Plate Combinations (e.g., Jewett nail, McGlaughlin nail, and side plate)

Used for both intracapsular and intertrochanteric fractures.
Problems with their use:

* *Same as tri-flanged nail*
* *The nail-side plate junction is an area subject to bending stress and may undergo fatigue failure of the metal*

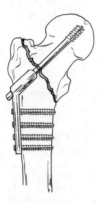

FIGURE 7.18.
Use of compression screws and side plate.

Compression Screws and Side Plate

Examples include Richards screw, the Zimmer compression screw, and the dynamic hip screw. They are used for both intracapsular and intertrochanteric fractures. When used to stabilize femoral neck fractures, some surgeons use an additional pin or a small screw to provide rotational control. When used to fix intertrochanteric fractures with extension into the proximal shaft, stability may be maintained by additional interfragmentary screws or cerclage wires. The function of the screw is to provide "dynamic compression" with weight bearing and/or resorption.

Problems with the use of compression screws and the side plate:

- *Cut out of screw in osteoporotic bone*
- *Screw may bind with weight bearing and may not slide in the barrel*
- *Side plate may not be snug on femur*
- *Long-barrel side plate may prevent impaction of intertrochanteric barrel*
- *Short-barrel side plate may allow lag screw to pull out*
- *Fatigue failure: may cause bending deformity or breakage at the junction of the barrel and side plate*

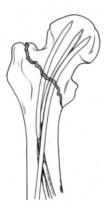

**FIGURE 7.19. Use
of Enders nails.**

Enders Nails

These are long flexible rods inserted at the distal femoral condyle and passed upward into the femoral head and neck.

Problems with their use include:

- *Knee pain: common from irritation of nails at the knee*
- *Nail cut out or penetration through osteoporotic bone of the femoral neck*

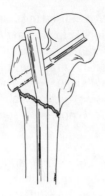

FIGURE 7.20.
Use of Zickel device.

Zickel Device

This is a combination of an intramedullary rod and a triflanged nail used for stabilization of subtrochanteric fractures and pathologic fractures of the proximal femur. The problem with its use is that the technically more difficult tri-flanged nail may penetrate the cortex of the femoral neck.

REFERENCES

Harley, J. D., L. A. Mack, and R. S. Winquist. "CT of acetabular fractures: Comparison with conventional radiography," *Am. J. Radiol.* 138:413–417 (1982).

Letournel, E. "Acetabulum fractures: Classification and management," *Clin. Orthop.* 151:81–106 (1980).

Young, J. W. R., A. R. Burgess, R. J. Brumback, and A. Poka. "Pelvic fractures: value of plain radiography in early assessment and management," *Radiology* 160:445–451 (1986).

8

KNEE INJURIES

INTRODUCTION

Many serious injuries to the knee region affect the ligaments and cartilage in or near the knee joint. These injuries, of course, are not directly visible on routine radiographs unless bony fragments are avulsed. The fractures and dislocations that occur in this area are less common than soft tissue injuries and present a challenge in treatment for the orthopedic surgeon. If the fractures involve the articular cartilage of the knee, there is the possibility that secondary degenerative arthritis will develop if the injury is not reduced and is held in an anatomic position. Also, fractures in the area can lead to a stiff knee, especially if there are fractures above and below the knee joint, i.e., a "floating knee" (Blake and McBryde, 1975). Nonunion is an additional problem if the treatment fails.

FRACTURES OF THE DISTAL FEMUR

Supracondylar fractures may have an intraarticular extension, which complicates the treatment and makes the need for anatomic reduction more important (Neer, 1967). There is controversy in orthopedic treatment regarding whether these injuries should be handled closed or with open reduction and fixation. There are difficulties in obtaining and maintaining reduction. Restoration of function is a problem, especially with intraarticular fractures. Operative reduction and internal fixation offer the best chance for healing, but often involve complicated surgical reconstruction. Many times, the medial portion of the fracture is slow to heal and may allow progressive varus deformity to develop. Bone grafting of the medial side is commonly done to try to avoid this.

Complications

- *Nonunion*
- *Malunion (angulation or rotation)*
- *Infection (from open injury or open treatment)*
- *Vascular injury to the superficial femoral or popliteal artery*
- *Fat or blood clot embolism*

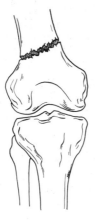

FIGURE 8.1.
Supracondylar
fracture.

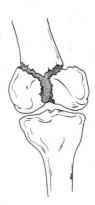

FIGURE 8.2.
Y-shaped inter-
condylar frac-
ture.

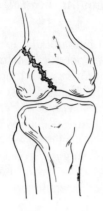

FIGURE 8.3.
Oblique single
condyle fracture.

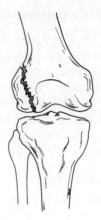

FIGURE 8.4.
Sagittal fracture.

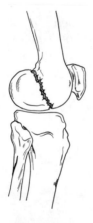

FIGURE 8.5.
Coronal frac-
ture.

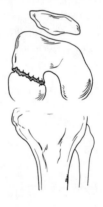

FIGURE 8.6.
Coronal oblique.

Radiographic Examination

Oblique views are helpful for intraarticular fractures in identifying the extent of displacement of the condylar fracture. One should always look for femoral neck fractures or patellar fractures if there is a mid- or distal femoral fracture from a "dashboard" injury.

FRACTURES OF THE PROXIMAL TIBIA AND THE TIBIAL SHAFT

Several classification schemes are in vogue for fractures involving the tibial plateaus, but the main descriptive components that the radiologist should be aware of are the following:

- *Undisplaced*
- *Local depression of the joint surface*
- *Vertical split*
- *Vertical split plus depression*
- *Bicondylar*
- *Plateau plus proximal tibial shaft*

As in the distal femur, treatment is controversial regarding closed or open methods for both intra- and extraarticular fractures. Criteria for internal fixation include depression of a plateau or separation of a fragment. Usually fractures with more than 5–7 mm of intraarticular displacement are treated with operative reduction and internal fixation. Fixation is often a buttress plate placed medially or laterally. When there has been significant depression of the articular surface, a corticocancellous graft may be placed under the subchondral bone for support after it has been elevated.

Complications

- *Varus or valgus angulation of depressed plateau fractures*
- *Angulation of shaft fractures*
- *Anterior or posterior compartment syndrome in the calf*
- *Nonunion*
- *Infection*
- *Posttraumatic arthritis*

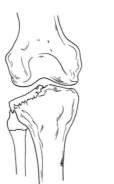
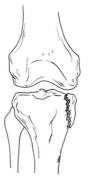

FIGURE 8.7.
Depressed tibial
plateau fracture.

FIGURE 8.8.
Split tibial plateau
fracture.

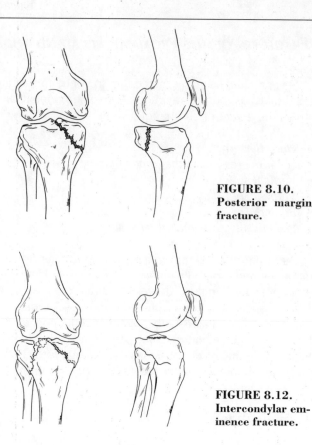

FIGURE 8.9.
Condylar fracture.

FIGURE 8.10.
Posterior margin
fracture.

FIGURE 8.11.
Comminuted bi-
condylar fracture.

FIGURE 8.12.
Intercondylar em-
inence fracture.

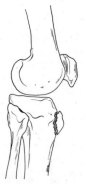

FIGURE 8.13. Fracture of the tibial tubercle.

The "lateral capsular sign" or Segond fracture is a small avulsion
fracture of the lateral edge of the tibial plateau. It is caused by rotation and
varus stress, usually as a result of a fall. It is almost always associated with
a tear of the anterior cruciate ligament and/or the menisci.

Radiographic Features

As in the distal femur, oblique views may be helpful both to identify subtle plateau fractures and to check angulation or depression. Tomography or computed tomography is sometimes used to look at the surface of the tibial plateaus if internal fixation is contemplated or a better assessment of displacement is required.

FRACTURE OF THE PROXIMAL AND MIDDLE FIBULA

Fractures of the proximal fibula are important because of associated injuries, such as fractures of the ankle with tear of the interosseous membrane (Maisonneuve fracture), injury to the peroneal nerve, or injury to the anterior tibial artery. There are three mechanisms of injury: direct blow, twisting injury to the ankle, and varus stress to the knee. Jumping can cause a twisting injury with anterior dislocation of the fibular head (parachute jumper's dislocation). A direct blow can cause posterior dislocation of the head (horseback rider's knee) or fracture of the proximal shaft (bumper fracture). Fractures of the fibular shaft usually heal without difficulty. However, if a fibular fracture heals before a tibial fracture at the same level, the fibula may prevent the necessary impaction at the tibial site, leading to tibial nonunion.

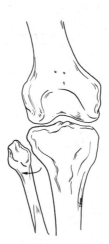

FIGURE 8.14.
Posterolateral dislocation of the proximal fibula.

PATELLA FRACTURE

These fractures occur either by direct blow or by avulsion of the quadriceps muscle or the patellar tendon. Patterns of fracture that are described include osteochondral, comminuted (stellate), transverse, oblique, vertical, and avulsion of the superior or inferior margin. Osteochondral fractures are frequently occult with patellar dislocation and are associated with hemarthrosis. They may be problematic, as radiographs may not reveal intraarticular fragments. If the clinical picture suggests significant retropatellar damage with an effusion, arthroscopy is frequently indicated.

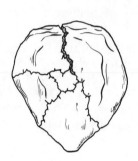 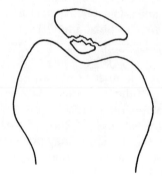

A. Comminuted fracture.   B. Osteochondral fracture.

FIGURE 8.15.

DISLOCATIONS AND LIGAMENTOUS INJURIES OF THE KNEE

With dislocation of the knee joint, vascular injury is common. Arteriography may be required to determine the presence of intimal tear of the popliteal artery or other arterial damage.

Acute dislocation of the patella is usually in a lateral direction and may be associated with hemarthrosis or an osteochondral fracture. Chronic subluxation or dislocation of the patella is most common in young females, and in this group the patella always dislocates laterally. Dislocation of the proximal tibiofibular joint can lead to unexplained pain and disability. Ligamentous injuries may have associated osteochondral fractures that are difficult to see.

REFERENCES

Blake R and A. McBryde. "The floating knee: Ipsilateral fractures of the tibia and femur," *South. Med. J.* 68:13 (1975).

Goldman, A. B., H. Pavlov, and D. Rubenstein. "The Segond fracture of the proximal tibia: A small avulsion that reflects major ligamentous damage," *Am. J. Radiol.* 151:1163–1167 (1988).

Hohl, M. "Tibial condylar fractures," *J. Bone Joint Surg.* 49A:1455–1467 (1967).

Neer, C. S., S. A. Grantham, and M. L. Ghelton. "Supracondylar fractures of the adult femur," *J. Bone Joint Surg.* 49A:592–613 (1967).

9

INJURIES TO THE ANKLE

INTRODUCTION

Injuries to the ankle occur from several mechanisms, which can produce specific patterns of injury on radiographs. Orthopedists take into account these mechanisms of injury when planning treatment. Therefore, it is important that the radiologist use terms in his or her report that describe the injury in adequate detail. A classification of ankle injuries was initially proposed by Dr. Lauge-Hansen in 1948, and this system, or a modification of it, is widely used by orthopedists.

Another classification system was developed by Danis, modified by Weber, and adopted by the Arbeitsgemeinschaft fur Osteosynthesefragen (AO) group. The types of fractures are as follows:

A. Supination injury with a fibular fracture below the level of the tibiotalar joint

B. Outward rotation of the talus with a fibular fracture at the level of the syndesmosis

C. Primarily an external rotation injury with a fibular fracture above the level of the syndesmosis

The following classification of ankle fractures and sprains was developed by Pettrone et al. (1983). There are five basic patterns of injury, and as the energy causing the injury increases, the damage produced progresses from ligament sprain to different combinations of fracture and ligament rupture or avulsion of bone fragments, depending on the direction and magnitude of the applied force. In this classification, the first word identifies the position of the foot at the moment of injury; the second word designates the direction of movement of the talus in relation to the leg as the injury occurs; and the last item is a grading number for the severity of the injury, depending on the number of structures injured.

Radiologists should become familiar with one of these classifications so that they can communicate with their clinical colleagues. The following descriptive terms are frequently used when describing ankle injuries. These include the position of the foot at the time of the injury and the direction of the deforming force.

Plantar flexion — movement of the foot distally or toward the plantar surface.

Dorsiflexion — movement of the foot proximally or away from the plantar surface.

Inversion — active turning of the sole of the foot to face inward.

Eversion — active turning of the sole of the foot to face outward.

Internal rotation — medial movement of the foot relative to the leg (big toe rotating toward midline of body).

External rotation — lateral movement of the foot relative to the leg (big toe rotating away from midline of body).

Adduction — the foot translates medially relative to the leg.

Abduction — the foot translates laterally relative to the leg.

Pronation — downward position of the medial border of the foot.

Supination — downward position of the lateral border of the foot.

SUPINATION-EXTERNAL ROTATION

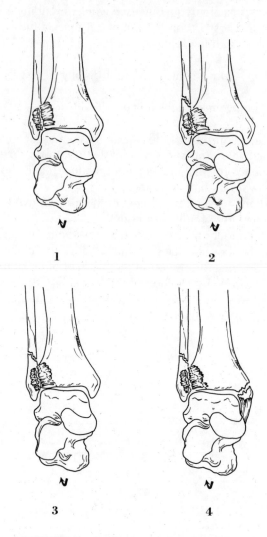

FIGURE 9.1. Supination-external rotation.

Grade

1. Rupture of the inferior anterior tibiofibular ligament
2. Spiral or oblique fracture of the lateral malleolus
3. Fracture of the posterior tibial margin or rupture of the posterior tibiofibular ligament
4. Rupture of the deltoid ligament or oblique fracture of the medial malleolus

SUPINATION-ADDUCTION

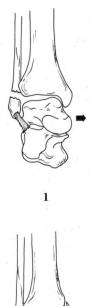

1

2

FIGURE 9.2. Supination-adduction.

Grade

1.   Transverse fracture of the lateral malleolus at or below the level of the ankle joint, or rupture of the talofibular ligament
2.   Nearly vertical fracture of the medial malleolus

PRONATION-EXTERNAL ROTATION

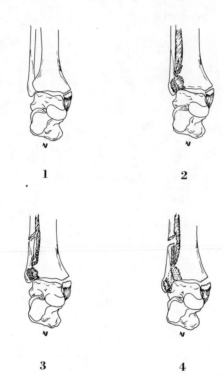

1   2

3   4

FIGURE 9.3. Pronation-external rotation.

Grade

1. Transverse fracture of the medial malleolus or rupture of the deltoid ligament
2. Rupture of the inferior anterior tibiofibular ligament and the interosseous ligament
3. Short spiral fracture of the fibula, typically located 3 in. proximal to the ankle joint but not infrequently more proximal
4. Avulsion fracture of the posterior tibial margin or rupture of the posterior tibiofibular ligament

PRONATION ABDUCTION

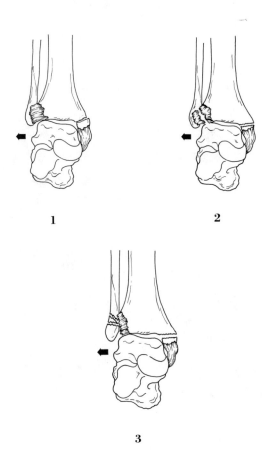

FIGURE 9.4.   **Pronation-abduction.**

Grade

1. Transverse fracture of the medial malleolus or rupture of the deltoid ligament
2. Rupture of both the anterior and posterior inferior tibiofibular ligaments with fracture of the posterior lip of the tibia
3. Oblique fracture of the fibula, generally just proximal to the ankle joint, often associated with displacement of a triangular fragment from the lateral surface of the fibula (interosseous ligament remains intact)

PRONATION-DORSIFLEXION

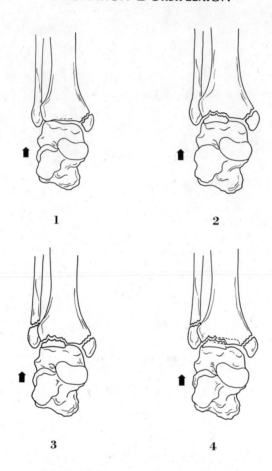

FIGURE 9.5. Pronation-dorsiflexion.

Grade

1. Transverse fracture of the medial malleolus
2. Avulsion fracture of the anterior articular margin of the tibia caused by dorsiflexion of the talus
3. Supramalleolar fracture of the fibula
4. Transverse fracture of the posterior lip of the tibial articular surface at the same level as the proximal margin of the large anterior tibial fragment

REFERENCES

DeSmet. A. A., F. W. Reckling, and G. R. McNamara. "Radiographic classification of ankle injuries," *J. Canad. Assoc. Radiol.* 33:142–147 (1982).

Lauge-Hansen, N. "Fractures of the ankle. IV. Clinical use of genetic Roentgen diagnosis and genetic reduction," *Arch. Surg.* 64:488–500 (1952).

Pettron, F., M. Gail, D. Pee, T. Fitzpatrick, and L. Van Herpe. "Quantitative criteria for prediction of the results after displaced fracture of the ankle," *J. Bone Joint Surg.* 65-A:667–677 (1983).

Rogers, L. "The ankle," in *Radiology of Skeletal Trauma*. (New York: Churchill Livingstone, 1982, pp 791-860).

10

INJURIES AND DEFORMITIES OF THE FOOT

INTRODUCTION

An understanding of foot anatomy, especially as it relates to the structure and alignment of the tarsal and metatarsal bones, is essential for adequate interpretation of X-rays of the foot. Trauma, degenerative change, or congenital anomaly can alter normal structure. A well-executed radiographic examination, interpreted correctly, will be the key to initial diagnosis and subsequent follow-up of many foot deformities.

The radiologist must be conversant with common descriptive terms that relate to foot alignment. The language is probably richer than it needs to be, and several terms are used synonymously for the same condition. The attachment to Latin terms seems to have remained stronger in the foot than elsewhere in the skeleton.

ROENTGEN TECHNIQUE

Usually AP and lateral views will suffice for the evaluation of foot deformity. These views must be taken weight bearing, with the tibial axis as vertical to the film as possible. In infants a person must press a board against the sole of the foot to simulate the weighted condition. This will allow the differentiation between supple and rigid deformities. In infants, the lateral film is taken with the hindfoot maximally dorsiflexed (in order to evaluate for equinus deformity). In tarsal coalitions an oblique, non-weight-bearing view may be helpful. Additionally the subtle talocalcaneal coalition may require either a PA tangential view of the calcaneus with the ankle dorsiflexed (Harris view), lateral tomography, or computed tomography in the coronal plane of the subtalar joint.

Following are definitions for normal and abnormal foot positions and the angular measurements of the various foot arches.

DEFINITIONS FOR FOOT POSITION

Valgus — Viewed from the front, the foot distal to the deformity is angulated away from the midline.
Varus — The opposite of valgus.
Inversion and **eversion** — Inversion is the turning of the sole of the foot to face inward. Eversion is the opposite. The talus remains fixed, and the other bones of the foot move in relationship to it. Most of the movement takes place at the subtalar (talocalcaneal) joint.
Adduction and **abduction** — The foot deviates toward the midline of the body in adduction; the opposite occurs in abduction. (In the foot these terms are sometimes used interchangeably with varus and valgus.)
Dorsi- and **plantarflexion** — This motion takes place primarily at the ankle joint with movement of the foot cephalad or caudad.
Supination and **pronation** — These are produced by a rotation of the calcaneus about the midline axis of the foot. In the foot, supination is a combination of adduction, inversion, and plantarflexion. Pronation is performed by abduction, eversion, and dorsiflexion.
Rotational axes of the foot — The ankle joint produces dorsi- and plantarflexion. The second axis is the subtalar joint. The subtalar joint produces mainly adduction and abduction but also a degree of dorsiflexion

and plantarflexion. In addition, the calcaneus can rotate on the talus about the foot's midline to produce inversion or eversion. When all of these subtalar movements occur simultaneously, they produce supination or pronation. The third significant rotational axis in the hindfoot is the transverse tarsal joint, which is formed by the articulation of the talus on the navicular and the calcaneus on the cuboid. These joints contribute to inversion/eversion and abduction/adduction.

Longitudinal arches of the foot — In walking, the foot forms a tripod touching the ground at the heel, the fifth metatarsal, and the first metatarsal head. The medial longitudinal arch is much higher than the lateral, with the talus being the keystone between the anterior and posterior parts of the arch.

NORMAL ANGLES OF THE FOOT

The normal position of the talus and calcaneus on the lateral view is determined by visualization of the sinus tarsi, which appears as an oval area of decreased density above the projection on the medial-upper border of the calcaneus, called the sustentaculum tali, where the neck of the talus joins the body at its inferior surface. Complete visualization indicates a level subtalar joint.

The talus has no muscular attachments and maintains its position by ligamentous attachments with the tibia, fibula, and calcaneus.

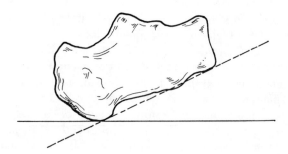

FIGURE 10.1. Calcaneal pitch. Normal = 20–30°. An index of the height of the foot framework.

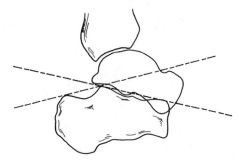

FIGURE 10.2. Boehler's angle. Normal = 28–40°. An indication of the integrity of the calcaneus. Fractures of the calcaneus will lower this angle and the calcaneal pitch.

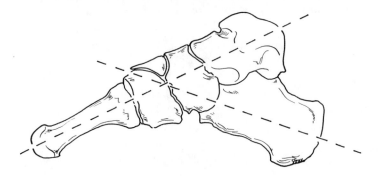

FIGURE 10.3. Talocalcaneal angle on lateral view. Normal = 25–40°. Normally, the midtalar line parallels the midshaft of the first metatarsal, except in infants where the talus is more vertical.

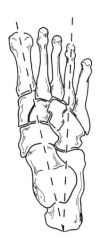

FIGURE 10.4. Talocalcaneal angle on AP view. Normal = 25–35° (lower in children). The talar line points to the first metatarsal, and the calcaneal line points to the fourth metatarsal. In heel varus, the angle is smaller; in the heel valgus, it is larger.

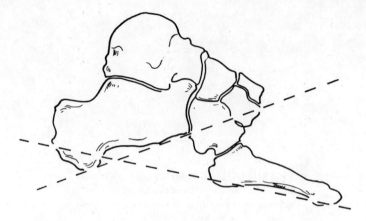

FIGURE 10.5. Lateral longitudinal arch. Normal = 150–175°. Inferior border of calcaneus to inferior border of fifth metatarsal.

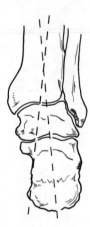

FIGURE 10.6. Heel valgus. From the rear the calcaneus normally slants outward 5–10°. This angle is difficult to view radiographically but can be inferred from the talocalcaneal angle on the AP view shown in Figure 10.4 (except in cases where a bone wedge has been removed surgically from the hindfoot).

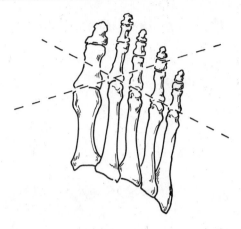

FIGURE 10.7. Angle of metatarsal heads. Normal = 140°.

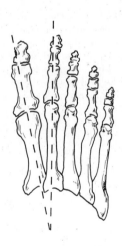

FIGURE 10.8. Inter-metatarsal angle. Normal = 5–10°.

FRACTURES AND DISLOCATIONS

Injuries to the Hindfoot

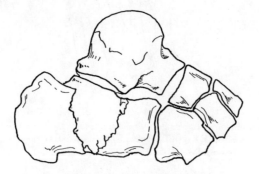

FIGURE 10.9. Fracture of the calcaneus. These are frequently comminuted and may extend through more than one of the compartments of the talocalcaneal joint. Usually Boehler's angle is decreased (q.v.). CT scan is helpful in showing the extent of subtalar joint involvement.

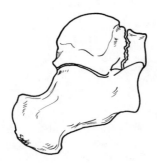

FIGURE 10.10. Fracture of the talus. If the fracture occurs in the neck of the talus, the blood supply to the dome of the talus may be interrupted, leading to osteonecrosis. Fractures in the coronal plane may be difficult to see, and lateral tomography will help.

Injuries to the Midfoot

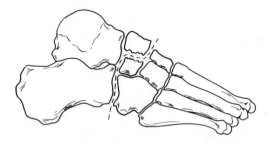

FIGURE 10.11. Chopart fracture-dislocation. This fracture separates the hindfoot from the midfoot. Navicular and/or cuboid fractures are common.

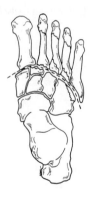

FIGURE 10.12. Lisfranc fracture-dilocation. This fracture separates the midfoot from the forefoot. Frequently there are fractures at the bases of the second, third, and fourth metatarsals. A comparison AP radiograph of the uninjured foot is useful in confirming lateral displacement of the fifth metatarsal relative to the cuboid.

Descriptions of Abnormal Foot Positions

Abnormal foot configuration may be congenital, developmental, post-traumatic, or secondary to neuromuscular impairment. The deformity may affect the entire foot or a segment, such as the hind-, mid-, or forefoot. The most severe deformities usually are congenital and involve the hindfoot.

Talipes — A deformity of the ankle and hindfoot *(tali* and *pes)* usually present at birth. Most commonly used to describe the condition known as *club foot* (q.v.).
Equinus — The calcaneus is plantarflexed and the heel cannot touch the ground with walking.
Calcaneus — The calcaneus is fixed in dorsiflexion (anterior end up).
Pes planus — Flatfoot. The longitudinal arch or calcaneal pitch is lower than normal. It is often associated with heel valgus or eversion, and pronation of the forefoot. It may be either rigid (spastic) or flexible (mobile). Spastic flatfoot is a painful condition associated with peroneal muscle spasm. The cause is a congenital synostosis between two of the bones of the hind- or midfoot. Alternatively the synostosis may be post-traumatic. These synostoses may be bony, fibrous, or pseudarthrodial. The joints involved may be:

> *talocalcaneal* (middle or posterior joints)
> *calcaneonavicular*
> *talonavicular* (occasionally)
> *calcaneocuboid* (rarely)
> *naviculocuneiform* (rarely)
> *naviculocuboid* (rarely)

Mobile flatfoot is developmental and the result of ligamentous laxity.
Pes cavus — A foot with a fixed high arch (increased talocalcaneal angle). It may be familial and associated either with calcaneovarus or calcaneovalgus. The severe forms are frequently associated with severe neuromuscular disease, e.g., Charcot-Marie-Tooth disease (progressive peroneal palsy).
Club foot — Talipes equinovarus. A severe congenital deformity consisting of equinus of the heel, inversion of the subtalar joint (heel varus and cavus), and metatarsus adductus. Complications of incomplete surgical treatment include residual rocker-bottom deformity due to failure to correct the hindfoot deformity and development of a flat-top talus. The post-club-foot rocker-bottom differs from the isolated form in that the talus is not vertically angulated in the former.
Rocker-bottom foot — Congenitally plantarflexed (vertical) talus. The heel is in equinovalgus and the arch is flat. It is also called *pes convex*. The navicular is dislocated dorsally on the plantarflexed talus.

Metatarsus adductus (varus) — Congenital inversion of the forefoot. Usually the first metatarsal is longer than the second.

Metatarsus atavicus — Congenital deformity with abnormally short first metatarsal.

Metatarsus latus — Congenital deformity with abnormally wide forefoot.

Metatarsus primus varus — Medial deviation of the first metatarsal shaft. Frequently seen with hallux valgus, bunion deformity, and atavistic first cuneiform (slanted metatarsal-cuneiform joint).

Bunion — Painful exostosis and soft tissue thickening on the medial aspect of the first metatarsal head. Associated with hallux valgus.

Dorsal bunion — Exostosis and soft tissue thickening due to flexion deformity of the first metatarsal phalangeal joint.

Bunionette — Varus deformity of the fifth toe with changes at the fifth metatarsal phalangeal joint similar to bunion deformity.

Morton's short first toe — An abnormally short first metatarsal which places stress on the second metatarsal, and the sesamoids under the head of the first metatarsal.

Hallux valgus — Acquired deformity, more common in women. The first toe deviates laterally at the metatarsal phalangeal joint. It usually is associated with metatarsus primus varus and planovalgus foot.

Hallux rigidus (limitus) — A painful, stiff first metatarsal phalangeal joint with osteoarthritis.

Hallux malleus — Hammertoe deformity of the great toe.

Hallux flexus — Flexion deformity of the interphalangeal joint of the great toe.

Hammer toes — Hyperflexed proximal interphalangeal joints of the second to fifth toes. All flexion deformities of the toes are commonly called hammer toes.

Claw toes — Hyperextended metatarsal phalangeal joints and hyperflexed interphalangeal joints. These may be associated with pes cavus or neuromuscular imbalance.

Mallet toes — Hyperflexion of the second to fifth distal interphalangeal joints.

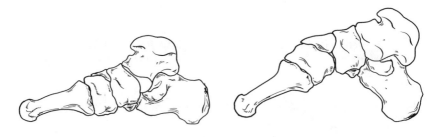

FIGURE 10.13. Pes planus.   **FIGURE 10.14. Pes cavus.**

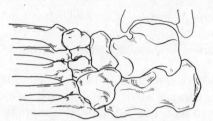

FIGURE 10.15. Club foot.

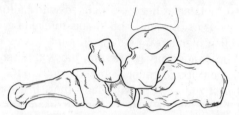

FIGURE 10.16. Rocker-bottom foot.

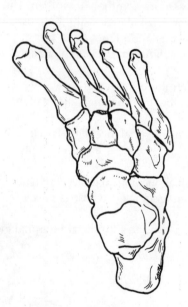

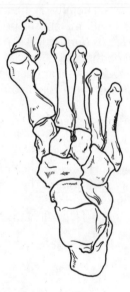

FIGURE 10.17.   Metatarsus adductus.

FIGURE 10.18. Metatarsus primus varus.

REFERENCES

Berquist, T. H., Ed. *Radiology of the Foot and Ankle.* (New York: Raven Press, 1989).

Blauvelt and Nelson, Eds. *A Manual of Orthopaedic Terminology.* (St. Louis: C. V. Mosby 1981).

Freiberger, R. L., A. H. Hersh, and M. O. Harrison. "Roentgen Examination of the Deformed Foot," *Semin. Roentg.* 5:(4):341–353 (1972).

Meschan I. "Radiology of the Normal Foot," *Semin. Roentg.* 5(4):327–340 (1972).

11

CLASSIFICATION OF VERTEBRAL FRACTURES ACCORDING TO MECHANISM OF INJURY

THORACOLUMBAR INJURY AND THE THREE-COLUMN CONCEPT

A review of thoracolumbar injuries by Denis has led to the development of a three-column concept that is now widely accepted. Radiologists should have a basic understanding of this when describing thoracolumbar injury patterns. The three columns are

Anterior — the anterior half of the vertebral body and intervertebral disc, and the anterior longitudinal ligament
Posterior — the posterior bony elements, interspinous ligament, capsular ligaments, and ligamentum flavum
Middle — the posterior longitudinal ligament, posterior part of the vertebral body, and posterior part of the anulus fibrosis.

The "middle" column was described separately from the traditional anterior and posterior structures because it is critical in the assessment of stable vs. unstable injuries. Failure of this middle column occurs in association with concomitant anterior or posterior column injury. It thus reflects an unstable injury (present or potential) and possible injury to neural elements.

CLASSIFICATION OF SPINAL INJURIES

Spine injuries result from either direct or indirect trauma. The bony injury will vary depending on the bone quality, type and magnitude of force, and associated soft tissue (ligament) injury.

Spinal fractures can be grouped as minor or major. Minor injuries are articular process fracture, transverse process fracture, spinous process fracture, and pars interarticularis fracture. Major injuries include compression fracture, burst fracture, distraction injuries, and fracture dislocations.

A classification of spinal injuries based on the major direction of the force applied follows.

COMPRESSION INJURY

Compression injury results from excessive axial load. The most common are the wedge fractures seen in osteoporotic bone. However, with greater force, the damage can be more than just trabecular compression. In all true compression fractures, the middle column remains intact and the fracture is stable. When the line of compression force passes anterior to the center of the disc, a flexion force is added to the axial load and a more complex fracture pattern, which is potentially unstable, develops.

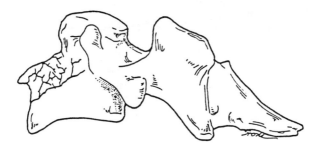

FIGURE 11.1. Compression (wedge) fracture.

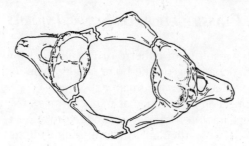

FIGURE 11.2. Jefferson fracture of C-1.

FLEXION INJURY

This is the most common mechanism for spinal fracture. This pattern is frequently seen at the thoracolumbar junction. Damage to the posterior elements is very unlikely (anterior column injury). Flexion fractures are usually stable and are not associated with a neurologic deficit. If the fracture demonstrates more than 50% loss of height and/or involves more than one vertebral body, there is a higher risk of posterior injury, progressive kyphosis, pain, and neurologic involvement. Chronic instability and kyphosis are most likely at the thoracolumbar junction.

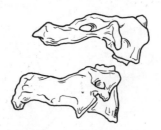

FIGURE 11.3. Anterior fracture-dislocation of the odontoid process.

A. Type I

B. Type II

C. Type III

FIGURE 11.4. Types of odontoid fracture.

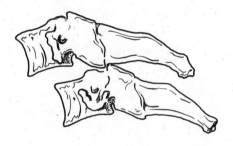

FIGURE 11.5. Bilateral locked facets.

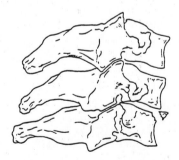

FIGURE 11.6. Teardrop fracture of the anterior margin of the vertebral body. (In some cases may be due to extension injury.)

BURST FRACTURE

The burst fracture with a flexion component and comminution of the vertebral body often has posterior element injury as well. CT scan will show disruption of the anterior and middle columns, and frequently of the posterior column. The disruption of all three spinal columns renders this type of fracture inherently unstable.

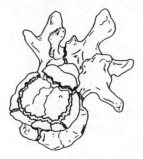

FIGURE 11.7. Burst fracture.

DISTRACTION INJURY

This is a result of deceleration injury with the pelvis fixed. A distraction force is applied to the spine with injury usually between L-1 and L-4 ("seat belt fracture"). The exact injury pattern is variable. A fracture can be "all bone" (the classic Chance fracture), purely soft tissue disruption, or a combination. Neurologic injury is rare (<5%). The true Chance fracture is usually stable because of the impaction of bony surfaces and heals rapidly. However, distraction injuries that disrupt the intervertebral disc and/or posterior ligaments are potentially very unstable and may displace, causing neurologic damage. Stabilization is required in these injuries to prevent displacement. Both the posterior and middle columns fail from the distraction. If the anterior column collapses, this becomes a fracture-dislocation injury.

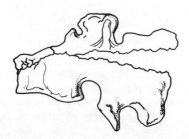

FIGURE 11.8. Distraction injury.

ROTATIONAL INJURY

Flexion with rotation can produce the unilateral locked facet injury of the cervical spine. Typically the upper vertebral body is displaced anteriorly 25% on the body below. Similarly, a twisting injury can occur between T-10 and L-1. (The ribs resist torsion above this, the lumbar facets below.) Whereas flexion alone rarely causes lateral/posterior column injury, flexion with rotation may often be associated with unstable injuries and neurologic damage, which is seen in 60–70% of all thoracolumbar fracture-dislocations.

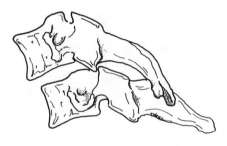

FIGURE 11.9.   Unilateral locked facet.

LATERAL BENDING INJURY

This may cause a lateral wedge fracture (fairly uncommon). Usually these are stable fractures and are not associated with a neurologic deficit. Lateral flexion is the presumed mechanism for uncinate process fracture in the cervical spine.

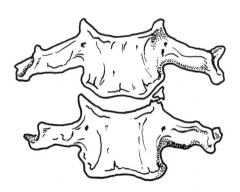

FIGURE 11.10.   Uncinate process fracture.

SHEAR INJURY

Shear or translational stress may cause injury with severe displacement with or without bony injury. The incidence of neurologic injury is very high, and these fractures are highly unstable. The goal of treatment is to reduce and restore stability.

EXTENSION INJURY

Hyperextension injuries are common in the cervical spine yet are unusual in the thoracic and lumbar spine. Typical examples of extension injuries in the cervical spine are "whiplash" injuries and "hangman" fractures. In the lumbar spine, extension forces most often affect the pars interarticularis region of the mid- to lower lumbar vertebrae ("traumatic spondylolysis"). This may occur as an acute injury with a sudden fracture or may develop as a chronic problem associated with fatigue failure of the pars. This lesion is seen frequently in gymnasts, heavy weightlifters, and football players. Extension injuries are usually stable and are rarely associated with neurologic injury. However, true traumatic spondylolysis and that occurring in skeletally immature patients may progress to spondylolisthesis. Serial lateral X-rays and flexion-extension views are the best way to follow these injuries.

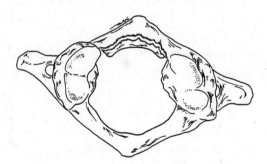

FIGURE 11.11. Horizontal fracture of the anterior arch of C-1.

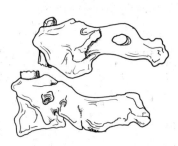

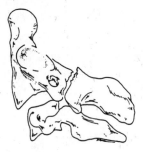

FIGURE 11.12.   Posterior fracture-dislocation of the odontoid process.

FIGURE 11.13.   Hangman fracture (traumatic spondylolisthesis of C-2).

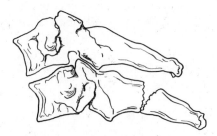

FIGURE 11.14.   Clay shoveler fracture (spinous process fracture).

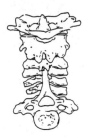

FIGURE 11.15.   Vertebral arch fracture due to compressive hyperextension (articular pillar, lamina, pedicle).

PRINCIPLES OF SPINAL INSTRUMENTATION

A variety of systems have been developed to treat disorders of the spine. The goals of instrumentation are

- *To improve stability*
- *To correct deformity*
- *To prevent progression of deformity*

The position of the implant is very important, because critical neurovascular elements must be protected. Radiographs in at least two planes are essential.

Note that in almost all instances these fixation devices are systems of "provisional stabilization" that depend upon a solid bony fusion for success. Without the support of spinal arthrodesis, these implants may demonstrate fatigue failure as a result of repetitive mechanical loads. Broken hardware in the spine may be evidence of a pseudarthrosis.

Wiring Techniques

Stainless steel wire is used to provide compression stability in the spine. It is usually placed around the bases of spinous processes and then tightened to compress the vertebral column.

Complications

- *Improper or unstable placement*
- *Cut out of wire through bone*
- *Breakage of wire occurring at the site of the twist/bend junction*

Sublaminar Wiring

Sublaminar wires have been used with several types of rod systems to provide segmental fixation points and to increase the stability of the implant construct. They must be passed underneath the lamina with great care.

Complications

- *Displacement causing dural tears and neurologic injury*
- *Wires cutting through the lamina*
- *Removal of the wires, which seems to carry a greater risk of dural injury than insertion*

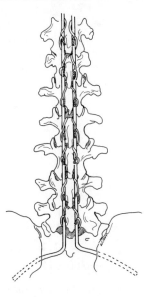

**FIGURE 11.16.   Sub-
laminar wiring.**

Segmental Spinous Process Wiring

This is a system of segmental wiring developed by Drs. Drummond and Keene and this is sometimes referred to as the *Wisconsin wiring technique*. Wires attached to buttons are passed through the bone at the base of the spinous process and then through a hole in the contralateral button to tighten down firmly on the base.

Complications

Although this system has markedly reduced the risk of dural tear, there is still a possibility of wire cut out and loss of fixation.

Facet Screws

Fixation screws are placed across the lumbar facet joints to provide stability for arthrodesis. Screw insertion is difficult as the amount of bone for purchase is limited and the tolerance for error is small.

Complications

- *Loss of fixation*
- *Facet fracture*
- *Malposition*
- *Nerve root irritation*

Harrington Rods

This system has become a "standard" of posterior instrumentation. It uses hook-fixation upon the lamina or transverse processes and either distraction or compression rods, or a combination of the two.

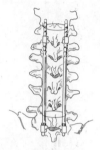

FIGURE 11.17.
Harrington rods.

Complications

Most common problems arise from the high stresses upon the hook-fixation sites. Hook malposition or cut out is a problem that occurs most frequently at the upper hook sites on distraction rods. If the small lock washer is not placed on the distraction rod below the upper hooks, the distraction may be lost and loose hardware may result. In spite of attempts to maintain the lordotic curve of the lumbar spine with Moe-modified Harrington rods, most of the fusions with posterior instrumentation at these levels will be relatively straight on a lateral X-ray, producing a condition known as *flat back syndrome,* which may be associated with severe pain.

Sacral Fixation

Special larger sacral hooks have been developed for stable seating in the sacrum. These are often used with the square-ended Moe distraction rod. This rod is contoured when inserted in an attempt to maintain the normal lumbar lordotic curve. The square end is commonly used with the Harrington system. They are subject to all of the failures mentioned above.

Knodt Rods

These are threaded rods with a central nut fixed to the rod and a "right hand-left hand" thread so that turns of the central nut can place a distraction force on the hooks at either end. A posterolateral spine fusion is usually performed. This system is most commonly used at L-4 to S-1.

Complications

- *Lamina fracture*
- *Hook migration or hook rotation resulting in loosening*
- *Hook irritation or erosion of the dura*

Luque Rods

Malleable smooth rods of variable length are contoured to fit a variety of spinal curves. Wires are passed underneath the lamina, then around the rods and twisted tight.

Complications

- *Sublaminar wires may cause dural tears*
- *Wires may loosen or break*

"Galveston" Modification of the Luque System

This procedure utilizes a special bend in the Luque rod that enables fixation to the sacrum. The rod is contoured in two planes so that the caudal end may be inserted at the posterior-superior iliac spine between inner and outer cortices of the ilium.

Complications

- *Penetration of the iliac cortex*
- *Rod loosening or breakage*
- *Entry into the sciatic notch with nerve irritation*

Cotrell-Dubousset

This is a posterior system of rods, hooks, crosslinks and pedicle screws. It was developed to provide correction of spinal deformity in the frontal, sagittal, and axial planes. Transverse rods placed at intervals create a coupled rectangle for stability. When used properly, the system is capable of treating a wide range of spine problems. This system is complex and proper placement of the hooks is critical.

Complications

- *Improper hook placement with loosening or impingement on the spinal canal*
- *Failure to place two transverse rods with resulting loss of stability of the system*

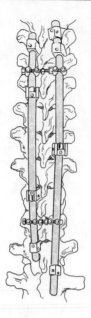

FIGURE 11.18.
Cotrell-Dubous-
set wiring.

Pedicle Screw Systems

Indications for the use of segmental pedicle fixation devices include

- *Spondylolisthesis*
- *Pseudarthrosis*
- *Degenerative instability*
- *Unstable fracture (i.e., burst fracture)*
- *Postdecompression instability*
- *Tumor-induced instability of the spine*

Contraindications for this include

- *Infection*
- *Highly osteoporotic bone*
- *Hypoplastic or absent pedicles*

A variety of systems using the pedicle screw as a spinal anchor have been developed. Accurate placement of screws into bone that will hold the anchor until fusion has occurred is important.

Complications

- *Malposition of the screws, which may traumatize major vessels*
- *Screws placed too laterally will lose purchase*
- *Screws too medial may irritate nerve roots*
- *Screws may fracture*
- *Screws may loosen*
- *Accelerated facet joint arthritis or instability*
- *Instability and listhesis*

Steffee Pedicle Screw System

This is a relatively rigid system of plates of variable lengths that fit over the pedicle screws to link segments of the spine together. The plates have slots to allow for distraction or compression.

Luque Plates

These were developed by Eduardo Luque, the same man who fashioned the Luque rods described above. The plates are less rigid than the Steffee plates and the notches for the pedicle screws will allow up to 15° of angulation at the screw-plate junction. Transverse bands on the plates are used to prevent the plates from spreading and loosening their hold on the screws.

Wiltse System

This system uses pedicle screws placed segmentally and then connected to a stainless steel rod by saddle clamps. With this system the rods may be contoured to match the deformity. When the goal of the procedure is spinal fusion, some authors feel successful spinal fusion is more likely if one accepts the deformity and fuses in situ. Either one or two rods can be used on each side of the spine, so that up to four rods may be used in cases where additional strength is a priorty.

Modular Spine Fixation System

This system uses pedicle screws with anchor holes at the top and bottom positions so that distraction hooks can be placed within. Intermediate screws are threaded and clamped onto the rod. The rod is called a *universal rod* and has the appearance of a Harrington distraction rod.

Internal Skeletal Fixation Systems

This system uses a Schanz screw as a pedicle anchor and then clamps the screw to a spinal fixation rod. It is used primarily as a distraction system, but the rod is threaded so that it has both distraction and compression capabilities. It is used primarily for thoracolumbar fractures. The pedicle anchor allows shorter instrumentation of the spinal segment.

Anterior Spinal Surgery

There has been increased attention to anterior spine surgery in recent years. The anterior approaches for treatment of deformity, spinal canal decompression, and fractures involving the anterior column have added a number of concerns to radiologic interpretation of spine films. The method of anterior spinal fusion usually includes vertebral disc excision with fusion. In cases of tumor the entire vertebral body may be resected. In such instances, the body will usually be replaced by strut grafts or formed blocks of methylmethacrylate and often some type of metal fixation device.

Complications

- *Postsurgical collapse with resorption of graft*
- *Infection*
- *Pseudarthrosis*

Dwyer/Zielke Instrumentation

Dwyer first introduced this system as a flexible cable that clamped onto screws placed in the vertebral body. Zielke modified the system by substituting a semirigid threaded rod. The Zielke system is formally named the *Ventral derotation spondylodesis* instrumentation. This system is used primarily for a thoracolumbar or lumbar scoliosis with a single curve pattern. Screws are placed all the way across the vertebral body to serve as bone anchors and are inserted from the convex side of the curve. The threaded rod is then inserted and nuts are threaded into the screw heads. Compression and derotation forces are applied, correcting the deformity, and the spine is fused, with the grafts placed slightly anterior in the disc spaces to enhance lordosis and to minimize kyphosis. The system utilizes a derotation device that also imparts lordosis to the construct, and this helps to avoid the "flat back" syndrome.

Complications

Pseudarthrosis: the failure of fusion rate has been fairly high. It is often seen in cases with broken rods or screws that have dislodged.

Anterior Plates/Screws

A number of anterior spinal fixation devices have been developed to anchor to the vertebral body with large cancellous screws. In addition to rod/cable systems such as the Zielke instrumentation, a contoured spinal plate and other rod systems are being used successfully for anterior stabilization. These plates are used to span two or three vertebral bodies.

Kaneda Device

This device is similar in principle to the Zielke instrumentation, but it uses two rods and a cross-clamp to provide more strength and rigidity. This system facilitates one-stage treatment of thoracolumbar lesions. Decompression is performed anteriorly; then, an anterior fusion is performed and supported by the device. Cancellous screws are used to anchor four-pronged plates to the lateral aspect of the vertebral body. Threaded rods link the vertebral elements together.

Complications

- *Pseudarthrosis*
- *Metal fatigue fracture*

REFERENCES

Aebi, M., C. Etter, T. Kehl, and J. Thalgott. "The Internal Skeletal Fixation System: A New Treatment of Thoracolumbar Fractures and Other Spinal Disorders" *Clin. Orthop.* 227:30–43 (1988).

Denis, F. "The Three Column Spine and Its Significance in the Classification of Acute Thoracolumbar Spinal Injuries," *Spine* 8:817–831 (1983).

Gehweiler, J.A., R. L. Osborne, and R. F. Becker. *The Radiology of Vertebral Trauma.* (Philadelphia: W. B. Saunders, 1980).

Rockwood, C.A. and D. P. Green. *Fractures in Adults.* (Philadelphia: Lippincott,1984).

INDEX